The Menopause and
M.E. (C.F.S.)

Gina Bailey

Gina Bailey Publishing (gina.bailey1@btinternet.com)

ISBN: 1481031805
ISBN-13: 978-1481031806

CONTENTS

Acknowledgments

ACKNOWLEDGMENTS

I would like to thank all the volunteers and their families who contacted me and were kind enough to share their experiences with me. Without their frank and honest comments it would not have been possible to write this book which I hope will offer other women with this illness guidance and reassurance for both them and their families as they encounter this period of change in their life

About this book

This book came about because of a lack of accessible information regarding ME and the menopause. I have suffered with ME since the age of 28 when I became ill after a case of pneumonia and although I had experienced a couple of bouts of illness (notably one in my early teens where I was ill on and off school frequently from an unknown cause over the course of a year) I had been a busy, active person.

I feel lucky that I had a supportive family and, although ill, I have spent very little time house or bed bound. I experienced the usual exhaustion, pain, brain fog and frustration that this illness causes with good spells where I have been 95% better before I over did things and had yet another relapse. I noticed changes though at the age of 41 where my night sweats seemed to increase (as did feeling hot during the day), an increase in fatigue, my periods became erratic, my mood swings even more so and my libido seem to all but disappear. When I reluctantly went to my doctor I felt that I was probably wasting his time but after a blood test he confirmed that I was entering the menopause. He advised that considering my age HRT would be beneficial for my bones, and restore my libido. I went home and after consideration decided that, although I had always planned to handle the menopause naturally I had also not expected it to happen for another 10 years so I would give it a try. Unfortunately for me within 4 weeks I had 5 cysts in one breast and was advised that it would be wiser not to continue with it.

It was at this point that I started to seriously research what to expect from both the menopause and my ME. I was concerned that not only was the menopause affecting my ME symptoms but also my relationships. I felt as if I was turning into a different person which was alarming. This was where I encountered problems because there seemed to be very little information anywhere. I could read about the menopause or ME but not both. I remembered reading an article somewhere about women with ME often having an early menopause some years before but couldn't find it anywhere. Finally I contacted Tony Britton at the ME Association and asked if there was any information because if not I was tempted to try and find the information and write something myself. He confirmed that there wasn't much information and that they were often asked about the subject and they would welcome anyone who wanted to look into the subject. The seed was firmly sown in my mind and soon it began to grow.

I started by compiling a questionnaire looking at how the menopause affected both women's ME symptoms, what they felt had worked or not and how their relationships had been effected. I contacted Tony again along with as many ME groups as I could asking for volunteers. Many of them seemed happy to help and advertised for me. Over the next few months I received requests by email for copies and replies started coming in. As it was quite a long questionnaire I stated that if they felt unable to complete it all that their story in their own words would be helpful and appreciated.

Alongside this I started trawling through forums looking for threads related to ME/CFS and the menopause, had conversations with women through Facebook and continued to read anything I could connected with either the illness or the menopause. As a hypnotherapist I already knew therapists who practiced reiki, massage, and reflexology, EFT, NLP and CBT so I was able to ask for their experiences. I had seen and experienced some of the benefits of alternative therapies both for myself and with clients I have seen.

This book is the result. I cannot claim that this is a large study of women, it isn't. I received just under 50 completed surveys and stories. Some had felt able to ask their partners to complete the questions I had asked. Some were uncomfortable answering questions relating to anything connected to their partners (be it emotional or physical). Those that did though were very open and frank. Perhaps some women thought the questions were too personal but I was interested in how the menopause affected their lives not just their physical symptoms. I am a big believer in the principle that the symptoms and limitations of ME are something which we have to manage and it doesn't just affect us but those around us. People around us, especially family, also have to adapt whether they like it or not. The menopause is yet another change and I was interested in how that impacted on relationships.

This book is not intended to be a substitute for obtaining advice from a qualified medical professional or practitioner who will know your personal medical history. Instead this book brings what information is available together in one place and can tell you of the experiences of others and what they feel has been of use.

For those who find it difficult concentrating I have tried to keep the chapters short so you can dip in and out when you feel up to reading. I hope it saves you having to trawl through various books and websites and piece the information together yourself.

I have made reference to the MEA survey carried out in May 2010 which looked at which treatments sufferers felt worked best for them and I would recommend that you take a look at this when deciding whether you feel this is appropriate for you. This study was looking at all ME sufferers (men and women) form all age groups. I have also looked at treatments for symptoms of the menopause and compared the two. Many of the symptoms of the menopause and ME are often similar and it is difficult to tell which is causing them. Also just as the symptoms and severity of ME vary dramatically from person to person so does the experience of the menopause. Consequently the effects of the menopause on our ME symptoms cannot be expected to be the same for everyone but hopefully this will shed some light on other women's experiences. Some women experienced a dramatic effect, others none at all. Some reported having made a full recovery although this was separate from the menopause. Personally I have found it extremely reassuring and comforting to know that I am not alone and that although the menopause may present us with fresh challenges and that for some at least it is not all negative.

ME – What is it?

For most of you choosing this book you will already know, and probably have experienced ME and the effects it can have. This short chapter is for those who don't so you can easily skip this chapter if you choose. ME stands for Myalgic Encephalomyelitis. It is also sometimes referred to as CFS (Chronic Fatigue Syndrome), PVFS (Post Viral Fatigue Syndrome) and CFIDS (Chronic Fatigue Immune Dysfunction Syndrome). It became known as yuppie flu in the 1980's due to the number of middle class higher achievers who seemed to be affected by it. Fortunately this description is not often used today. For the purposes of this book when I refer to ME or ME/CFS I am referring to all of these labels. There are no simple blood tests that can diagnose the conditions but the primary symptom is extreme mental and physical fatigue. It is usually triggered by an infection (usually viral), a period of extreme stress but can sometimes have a gradual onset.

This illness affects the body and brain function as well as the central nervous system. The degree of symptoms varies from those who are able to manage their conditions by carefully balancing their life and energy levels but can function almost normally to those who are unable to speak, swallow or walk. The major symptom is the prolonged recovery from activity. Typically a sufferer will experience a fluctuation of symptoms but the prolong recovery from any activity (physical or mental) can severely affect normal life.

Symptoms include

Extreme fatigue with exercise
Muscle fatigue, spasms and pain
Muscle weakness (often for days) after use

Joint pain

Headaches

Dizziness

Loss of concentration and short term memory problems (brain fog)

Flu like symptoms (reoccurring sore throat, enlarged or painful lymph glands)

Sleep disorders (vivid dreams/nightmares, sleeping too much, disturbed sleep)

Digestive problems

Poor temperature control (including night sweats, cold hands and feet, excess sweating)

Clumsiness

Balance problems

Feeling faint

Sensitivity to sound, tinnitus

Visual disturbances (blurring, feeling disorientated)

A grey pallor to skin (when suffering a relapse)

Easier to walk slowly than stand

Feeling disorientated

Poor bladder control

Chest pains

Depression and feeling over emotional (crying, mood changes)

Fluctuation of symptoms (frequent relapses followed by periods of feeling better)

With such a wide range of symptoms it is not surprising that it is difficult to diagnose or predict the varieties of ways in which this illness can impair your everyday life. That this illness seems to hit people who have generally been busy and active individuals is a common thread running through most articles concerning the subject. It can therefore be devastating for both the sufferer and their families when it strikes.

There are stories of people who have "recovered" from this illness but for the vast majority they have to learn to manage their illness and managing an illness that, by its nature can fluctuate from day to day, is no easy task. It is hard to explain just how exhausted you feel by doing a simple task because everybody gets tired. For someone to learn that this illness leaves you beyond tired takes time and understanding.

History of the menopause

It is only in the last 100 or so years that we have known about hormones and how they work. A lack of medical knowledge meant various myths evolved as an explanation of how the human body worked. These, when mixed with religious beliefs and views of women at this time, led to a major misunderstanding of the menopause. A large number of these negative attitudes still remain today despite our increased knowledge.

The monthly menstrual period was believed by some pagan and religious teachings to be a sign that the woman had a covenant with the devil. A woman's duty was to bear children and others saw the monthly bleed as nature's way of cleansing her body, ridding her of the impurities within her body. Women were seen to have outlived their usefulness when she reached the end of her reproductive years. The end of menstruation (the menopause) was proof that she was no longer able to contribute to the continuation of her husband's family line or to society in general.

The French physician, **de Gardanne**, first used the term 'menopause' in 1812. During this time experts had a trend of gaining medical and scientific understanding through examining bodily organs and fluids. This marked a move away from satanic accusations but did little for the understanding of the female anatomy. Women at this time were generally not living beyond their 40's or their reproductive years.

At this time women's organs were thought to make them emotional and unstable, and therefore inferior to men who were strong. In contrast women were considered hysterical. The word hysterical comes from the Greek word 'hystericus'. Hysteria was a description of women when something was wrong with the uterus. A hysterectomy (removal of the organs) was seen as the way to correct a woman's health.

During the late 1800-1900's psychiatry became more popular. People, especially women, were considered immoral and lacking proper judgment if they had any thoughts about intercourse other than reproduction. Women's neurotic tendencies did not help them. Victorians saw the menopause as a mysterious debilitating psychological condition. It was treated with mood altering tranquillizers, shock treatments and in some cases institutionalization. Life expectancy at this time was not usually above 48 and it was normal for women to give birth to approximately 8 children. The 'change of life' was believed to allow women's nervous system to become unhinged and to deprive them of their personal charm.

English lecturer and cultural researcher, Sally Shutterworth, describes in her writing the perceived relationship between women's menstrual cycles, circulation and mental health. This shows how doctors in the past believed that a woman's body controlled her mind and regulating a woman's period regulated her mental health.

Any changes in menstrual flow were believed to be a form of mental disorder. This was due to the belief that the physiological, emotional and mental states were interdependent. Due to the role of a woman's period in the circulating system of both the body and the mind it was also believed that strong emotions could cause menstrual problems or obstructions when blood could not escape through its usual route so this could in turn lead to insanity or even death. It was believed that irreparable psychological breakdown could be caused by blood flooding the brain without its usual path for leaving the body.

English physiologists Ernest Starling and William Bayliss discovered the first hormone in 1902. Modern science differentiated between oestrogen and progesterone around 1925 and would discover over the next decades how oestrogen can be used to deal with a variety of both physical and mental symptoms of the menopause. Modern HRT (hormone replacement therapy) is based on these findings.

Life expectancies increased and women were living longer but still women were subjected to ridicule and regarded as second class or less valued members of society. Social attitudes towards the menopause lagged behind the medical and scientific advances as generations went through 'the change' and lived beyond women from previous generations.

In March 2005 the NIH (National Institute of Health) issued a statement concluding that the menopause was a natural phase in a woman's life and NOT a disease to be treated or eliminated.

The Menopause – What is it?

The word menopause comes from the Greek words 'pausis' meaning cessation and 'men' meaning month. It literally means the 'end of cycle'. It is referring to a woman's menstrual cycles so it is when her menstrual cycle (i.e. her periods) ends. This is the end of the fertile stage of a woman's life. This is when the primary function of her ovaries reached permanent cessation. Basically it is simply when a woman stops menstruating. The average age for a woman to have her last period is 51.

To confuse the issue this time is divided further and these times will be referred to as peri-menopause, pre-menopause and post-menopause. This is because the technical time to reach the menopause is 12 months after your last period. Pre-menopause is the time leading up to your last period. Peri-menopause is the years leading up to post-menopause. This is when your hormone levels are changing and is a period of transition. It can cover from several years before your last period through until you are post-menopausal. Post-menopause years are the ones following the year after your last period. Clearly you do not know if you have had your last period at the time. You may have irregular or erratic periods for some time before the very last one. Many women refer to going through the menopause when technically they are going through the peri-menopause.

Early Menopause

There are several reasons for experiencing an early menopause. They are

- Surgery to remove you ovaries – you develop menopausal symptoms straight away

- Having radiotherapy to the pelvic area as treatment for cancer
- Some chemotherapy drugs that treat cancer may lead to an early menopause
- If you have had a hysterectomy (removal of the uterus) before your menopause. Although your ovaries will still produce oestrogen its rate will fall earlier. It may not be clear when you are in the menopause as you do not have periods after a hysterectomy but you may develop symptoms as your oestrogen levels fall.
- Hereditary early menopause can run in some families
- Sometimes no cause can be found

One of the reasons for starting to write this book was that I had read that there seemed to be a link between the women with ME experiencing an early menopause. After being told that my hormone levels showed I was "further into the menopause than you might think" at 41 I started trying to find some information about how to manage my ME through this stage and I could find very little.

First let's look at the definitions connected to the menopause.

Premature menopause
Premature menopause or premature ovarian failure (POF) is usually referred to as menopause under the age of 40, although according some sites suggest that in the developed world this should be before the age of 45. According to Menopause Matters website premature ovarian failure (POF) is estimated to effect 1% of women under 40 and 0.1% under 30.

Peri-menopause
There is a large degree of variation on when and how long this

occurs when researching this. Some suggest that it is around the age of 40 while others suggest it will last between 10 and 20 years. This is the time where our bodies go through the transition into the menopause. Some say it lasts until 12 months after your last period while others suggest it is few a years' either side of it. Whenever it occurs this is the time when you could start to experience mood swings, night sweats and hot flushes due to fluctuating hormone levels. You may also notice changes in your periods. They may shorten or not happen at all some months. Some books suggest that our peri to post menopause stage lasts from our mid 30's to our mid 50's and points out that this is a quarter of our lives.

Menopause
You are classed as being in the menopause when you have not had a period for 12 months. The average menopausal age in the UK is 51-52.

Post-menopause
This overlaps the final year of the peri-menopause and is after your periods have stopped. Symptoms in the majority of women will ease and stop as your hormone levels stabilize and your body adjusts to the new levels produced.

Early menopause and ME/CFS

"Many women with ME/CFS experience an early menopause, or a drop in natural oestrogen levels, while maybe still in their thirties." Dr Anne Macintyre – M.E. Chronic Fatigue Syndrome: A Practical Guide

"..many symptoms overlap, particularly vasomotor instability (hot flushes, night sweats, palpitations) which is due to the oversensitivity of the autonomic system. Consequently, the two conditions will interact to exacerbate one another." Dr Charles Shepherd – Living with M.E.

There is little information on how or if ME sufferers are more prone to an early menopause other than the odd mention in an article. The responses I received had several in their 30's, the majority in their 40's (average age of these was 47) and the least number in their 50's. This does put us entering the menopause slightly earlier although it depends whether the volunteers were classing the age of their menopause as when they first started getting symptoms or the specific time of 1 year since their last period.

SYMPTOMS AND TESTS

Tests

Women are born with a certain number of eggs cells and with age these decrease until there are only a few left around the age of 45-55. Follicle Stimulating Hormone (FSH) and Luteinising Hormone (LH) control the ovaries which become less and less responsive and produce less oestrogen. Oestrogen levels drop over time and it is the consistent low levels of oestrogen that causes the woman's periods to stop.

The common test used to diagnose the menopause checks for the levels of FSH and LH. This is because the drop in oestrogen and progesterone production during the menopause leads to an increase in FSH and LH. This can be done by a simple blood test.

Symptoms

Not every woman will experience all these symptoms of the menopause. In fact some women will experience no symptoms at all.

Common Symptoms are –

- hot flushes
- night sweats
- mood swings
- irregular periods
- loss of libido
- vaginal dryness
- fatigue
- sleep disorders
- difficulty concentrating

- memory lapses
- dizziness
- hair loss
- incontinence
- bloating
- allergies
- brittle nails
- changes in body odour
- feeling panicky
- depression and anxiety
- irritability
- weight gain
- headaches
- breast pain
- joint pain
- digestive pain
- problems with gums
- electric shocks and tingling extremities
- muscle tension and itchy skin
- osteoporosis

Menopausal symptoms and ME

Of the replies I received 20% said they had either no real symptoms either due to the fact that they were already on HRT prior to the menopause prescribed for their ME or that both the menopause and their ME started at about the same time making it difficult to distinguish between them. I have heard women say that you "would definitely know if you were having a hot flush and if you don't then it isn't one". The difficulty I have with this is that I personally know that I have been suffering from night sweats for 14 years and that my hormone levels meant I was not even peri-menopausal . These were purely down to my ME/CFS. If I was run down or going through a bad patch I would experience poor temperature control during the day and horrendous night sweats. I cannot tell the difference. I do get more during the day now and get them when I am relatively well. That is the only difference I can find.

Most of the symptoms listed for the menopause as the same or similar to ME. The main comments have concentrated on hot flushes which can be very draining. Draining someone who already has limited energy supplies can exacerbate existing symptoms. While some women have responded saying that the menopause has had a detrimental effect on their illness others have reported no change. Some actually feel better. The absence of monthly periods which have been regularly increasing their ME symptoms are seen as a blessing.

Here's what some ME sufferers replied when asked "How have the symptoms of the menopause affected your ME?"

"Increased dramatically fatigue and migraines (turned headaches into migraines), lowered already low libido, night sweats, sleep worsened, anxiety increased and low mood worsened"

"I felt like I was losing my mind. My symptoms of ME seemed to get worse. I had pain in my legs and back and was thrown back into stages of complete exhaustion. I was experiencing more brain fog and mood swings as well as night sweats (which increased and included hot flushes during the day). My stamina levels seemed non-existent."

"At the start of the menopause I had heavier more frequent periods with bad headaches and my energy levels and immune

function went down each time."

"My migraines, body aches and exhaustion became worse."

"I'm not aware that they have."

"I have all the traits of the menopause and ME, foggy brain, lack of concentration, bouts of mild depression, anxiety etc (which one is which I don't know)."

"Less energy, more anxious, deterioration in cognitive function (particularly short term memory)"

"I have wondered how much my ME has been exacerbated by the hot flushes as when I have relapses the flushes seem much worse. Or whether some of the flushes have been due to the ME and not the menopause, it's hard to tell."

"I'm not sure I have had any menopausal symptoms."

Allergies

There seem to be ongoing debate about whether allergies are a symptom of ME. While some people do suffer from allergies is seems unclear as to whether this is part of their illness or something else running alongside it. From the responses I have received there appears to a quite a number of women who are suffering from food allergies. This echo's the findings of the ME Associations survey in May 2010 which showed that more than half of those surveyed considered that their allergies were a major or minor symptom of their illness.

Often intolerances are describes are allergies. An allergy is described as an "over enthusiastic response by the immune system to factors which most people would regard as harmless". This is usually inherited or from birth. Intolerance is a heightened sensitivity that is subtle or minor or a new one. These are usually to fur or dander, pollen (or chemicals) and foods. An allergic reaction is usually quite quick when exposed to an item whereas intolerance can take longer (up to 24 hours) for symptoms to appear. They may also come and go, especially with food, if it is avoided for several weeks. You may have a reaction to something that can make you feel very unwell which is not necessarily an allergy but could be intolerance or sensitivity. I am not trying to trivialize intolerances because I know these can be very debilitating until you are able to identify and eliminate a substance from your diet or lifestyle. Intolerance to foods can be just as hard to live with as an allergy. To keep it simple I will refer to both of these as allergies during this chapter.

The triggers for allergies are usually diet, stress and hormone fluctuation. Some people will always experience problems caused by allergies but the main times when allergies can flare up in women are at puberty, menstruation, pregnancy and the menopause when their hormone levels are fluctuating. Allergies can flare up because the hormones and the immune system are connected therefore changes in one can produce changes in the other. Changes in hormones are thought to have an impact on the severity and number of allergies.

The common allergies are eczema, asthma, hives, hay fever and allergic shock. The symptoms can range from mild (rashes, sneezing, congestion and itchy eyes) to moderate (difficulty breathing and itchiness) and severe (vomiting, cramps diarrhoea, abdominal pain, swelling and confusion). Another symptom is migraines which can be debilitating. Allergies can usually be improved by making lifestyle changes, such as eliminating certain foods, avoiding contact with chemicals and being in the fresh hair. There are ranges of alternative medicines/therapies which can help (herbs, supplement and even acupuncture) or prescribed and over the counter treatments. The best form of management seems to be a combination of lifestyle changes and alternative medicines/therapies as many of the prescribed drugs have side-effects. Allergies are often treated with antihistamines and anti-inflammatory steroids which are not recommended for people with ME/CFS unless absolutely necessary.

Allergies can be inherited and the likelihood of having an allergy increases if your parents also have them. If neither parents' have allergies a child has a 15% chance of experiencing them but rises to 30% if one parent has them and 60% if both parents have them. While only 2% of adults and 8% of children have food allergies it is estimated that 45% of people have food intolerances.

Dairy and wheat, in particular, seem to be foods that can cause problems. Many people try to eliminate these from their diet at some time. It may be that your system is overloaded and simply having a break will be enough to sort the problem out. This could be due to fluctuations in both the immune system and your hormones. It can be difficult to distinguish between some illnesses such as IBS (Irritable Bowel Syndrome), inflammatory bowel disease or gastrointestinal obstructions. Coeliac disease is a condition where the sufferer has an adverse reaction to gluten. This is an auto-immune condition and not an allergy or intolerance.

There are tests which can determine whether you actually do have an allergy to a certain substance. Your doctor may be able to arrange for you to have either a skin or blood test. They may refer you to an allergy clinic. Not all areas have allergy clinics so you may have to travel. If you feel unable to wait or your doctor won't refer you there are a wide variety of companies who advertise offering to test for allergies. These vary is cost and offer to test everything including skin, hair, eyes, blood so it is always best to check that it is a reputable clinic performing the test. It is important to do your research as some private companies are better than others. Check how they test and what they are testing for before parting with your money. The NHS can provide you with a list of accredited allergy specialists.

An elimination diet can help you identify foods which cause you to have a reaction or are intolerant to. This involves keeping a strict diary where you record everything that you eat and your reactions. You eliminate foods for a certain period and then reintroduce the foods and record their effects. There are plenty of books and information on how to do this but I will add a note of caution. For someone suffering from an illness that leaves them exhausted any major change to their diet may not be wise. It is best to discuss this with your doctor first. You may feel unwell and suspect you have an allergy or intolerance but you do not want to trigger a relapse by suddenly changing your diet. If you do decide to follow an elimination diet please be aware of hidden ingredients. You will be amazed what you will discover, many paracetamol actually contain lactose, so check your medication.

Anaphylactic shock (anaphylaxis)

A severe and life threatening reaction is anaphylactic shock (anaphylaxis). This is a severe and sudden onset of symptoms which progress rapidly. It affects the circulation of the blood, breathing and the airways. This is treated by injecting insulin and people who have are severely allergic may be prescribed an auto-injector to carry with them as a precaution.

1 in 1300 people in England will develop symptoms of Anaphylaxis as some time during their life.

1 in 12 will go on to experience another episode

20-30 people die from Anaphylaxis each year in the UK

This type of reaction is slightly more common in women and people with other allergic conditions such as asthma and otopic eczema. Most people experience no long-term complications and make a full recovery if treated quickly with adrenaline.

Signs of anaphylactic shock are difficulty breathing, dizziness, skin changes (raised red rash or itchy skin) and swelling of certain body parts such as the lips, hands and feet. Common triggers are nuts, fish, eggs, milk, bee and wasp stings, and medication. If you suspect someone is going into anaphylactic shock then you should phone 999 immediately. Always check to see if they are wearing an allergy alert bracelet which will say if they have an auto-injector. If they have this should be injected into the thigh muscle and held in place for 10 seconds.

Allergies, ME and the menopause

As I have said our hormones and immune system are interwoven and interconnected. As we go through the menopause our hormone levels fluctuate and can cause allergies to flare up in the body. I have found personally that I get skin rashes when I am having a bad period with my ME. This has got worse at times when I am experiencing menopausal symptoms and I do think this is linked. There is very little evidence to support this although many other sufferers feel that their ME and allergies are link and/or interact with each other. However the MEA survey does indicate that there some sufferers do experience new allergies as well as intolerance to alcohol when developing this illness. It also shows from their responses that over 50% found an improvement when using allergy treatments with only 3.6% reporting this treatment has made them worse. Therefore I would suggest that trying allergy treatments has a much higher chance of improving your symptoms than causing you to feel any worse. It is always best to get an opinion from an expert and keep your doctor informed of any treatment to ensure it has no effects on any existing medication.

Yet again balancing your hormone levels may help. Our bodies are dealing with an illness which can heighten our sensitivity as well as hormone changes which can add to that. Restricted diets are not generally recommended for people with ME so any elimination diet should be handled very carefully. It is best to discuss this with your doctor first. A system which is already under strain from illness may not react well to a sudden change of diet and that must be balanced against the benefits of being able to avoid the symptoms of an allergy or intolerance. It is also best to try any elimination diet when you are feeling well and your illness is stable so there is less possibility of confusing any symptoms of your ME with any reactions you might experience to foods.

Some of the responses I received were from people who experienced a wide range of allergies and intolerances which had taken a long time to diagnose. The treatments that worked seemed to vary as much as their symptoms. It is reasonable to find that, whether the initial cause of the allergy or intolerance was related to their ME, trying to manage their lifestyle to avoid the food or substance causing the problem had improved their health. It had not "cured" their ME but they were able to manage it better. Changing your lifestyle to avoid the substance or food that causes a reaction can make the difference between feeling ill and being able to cope on a day to day basis.

It is important to be vigilant when checking food labels and not being afraid to ask how food is prepared when eating out especially if your reaction is severe. It may be that after a break you are able to start reintroducing that food or tolerate a small amount. For other people, once they have discovered the cause, they prefer to reassess their diet for life rather than ever endure the symptoms again. It can require willpower though as, ironically; you often actually crave the food that provokes a reaction.

Some pub/restaurant chains now provide information on their websites listing dishes that contain lactose, nuts, and other common triggers. They sometimes will go so far as to list if they are prepared in the same area so you can be aware of any risks of transference or trace of that ingredient.

"Suddenly I was unable to tolerate many of the foods I had previously eaten successfully. Apart from the usual culprits (cheese, chocolate, red wine) white flour was a particular problem and just one bite of bread would cause my head to reel with vertigo."

"I found that I had less tolerance to alcohol and certain foods would trigger migraines."

"I was completely intolerant of caffeine and had irregular heartbeats with just one cup of tea"

Appearance

Among the replies I received there was little mentioned about problems connected with appearance with the exception of a few more wrinkles and one lady who experience severe problems with body odour, however I should point out that this was one area which I did not ask about specifically. I have covered how this affects women in general going through the menopause and not specifically those with ME.

Hair Loss

This can be a thinning of or loss of hair on your head or anywhere on your body. There may be thinning of the pubic hair. Hair may become more brittle and drier.

What causes this?

The most common hair problem for women is estrogenic alopecia. The hair follicles need oestrogen and the changes are due to a deficiency in the body.

Treatments

Diet affects the rate of hair growth and improving overall health will be beneficial. Try to minimize damage by avoiding twisting and pulling hair. If you are having severe problems consult your doctor.

Brittle Nails

This can show as nails that split or chip easily, changes in colour, ridges on the nails, curling of the nail around the finger, having a sunken appearance and a feeling of dryness.

What causes this?

Again this is primarily down to fluctuating hormones, Oestrogen helps regulate water retention in the body and as its level decreases it can lead to dehydration which can show as brittle, dry nails that crack. Other causes can be poor circulation, anaemia, infection, liver disease, thyroid problems and deficiency in vitamin C, calcium, folic acid, protein, iron and fat, and stress which can weaken nails and slow growth. If you have other symptoms and you have a discolouration or split nails consult your doctor as this can be a sign of a more serious condition

Treatments

Lifestyle and diet changes can help. Ensuring that you have a good diet rich in vitamins and minerals will help. Nail growth can be improved by eating almonds as they contain fatty acids, as few as 6 a day can produce visible results.

Skin

Women can experience acne, thinning of the skin, pigments and wrinkles during the menopause. Many women also experience itchy skin. Some may also develop allergies and eczema flare ups.

What causes this?

It is thought that increased androgen levels during the menopause increase acne levels. Lower oestrogen levels slow the production of natural skin oils and the ability to retain moisture. Collagen in the skin (a fibrous protein that provides the skin and other tissues with resilience, support and strength) decreases with oestrogen levels as it is responsible for stimulating collagen production. This decrease is quickest in the peri-menopause (before the menopause). Other causes can be the side-effects of medication/drugs (or withdrawal symptoms), diabetes, skin cancer, fungal infections, hypothyroidism, herpes and vitamin deficiency. Fluctuations in hormone (which is also linked to the immune system) can cause the body to be hypersensitive and reactions occur such as eczema and allergy flare ups.

Treatments

Adult acne (usually on the lower face) rarely responds to teen acne treatments. To improve your skin you should increase your water intake to keep yourself hydrated. Healthy skin needs your diet to include enough vitamin B. It is also advisable to increase your levels of Omega-3 fatty acids. This can be found in foods such as walnuts, sardines, salmon, flaxseeds, soy and fortified eggs. Take shorter warm showers rather than hot ones as hot water has a harsh drying effect on the skin. Moisturize your skin and choose non-irritant gentle soaps. Apply a broad-spectrum, quality sunscreen. Trying to avoid over exposure to the skin will also help with your management of itchy skin. Again a healthy lifestyle will help and trying to balance hormones, which is the underlying cause, will have the best effects.

Body Odour

Apocrine glands in the underarms groin and near the hair follicles produce sweat which contains fatty compounds, bacteria then feeds on this in the skin. This forms an odour from the chemical reactions, fatty acids, waste products and ammonia. Excess sweating from hot flushes and night sweats can lead to a change in body odour.

What causes this?

The main cause is hormone fluctuations. Body temperature is controlled by the hypothalamus, as levels drop this can send a false message (that we are overheating) so it then increases sweat production, resulting in body odour.

Treatments

Diet and stress can also affect this, as can certain diseases. Seafood (particularly oysters) and nuts both contain zinc and magnesium which can help banish body odour. Non-breathable and synthetic fabrics can collect sweat and increases body odours. Try to wear natural fabrics such as cottons instead.

An interesting fact – The body odour of vegetarian's is more attractive than meat eaters according men and women in a blind study.

Cognitive problems

This can include difficulty concentrating and memory lapses. On a day to day basis this can manifest itself as forgetfulness, losing your train of thought, disorientation and an inability to concentrate on tasks, both everyday and complex ones.

What is the cause?

Again this is due to hormonal fluctuation. Neurotransmitters in the brain regulate cognitive functions including the ability to concentrate and memory. It has been shown that ACETYLCHOLINE and NOREPINEPHRINE regulate cognitive abilities which decrease if there is a shortage in these neurotransmitters (which leads to a difficulty in concentrating). Oestrogen stimulates blood flow to the brain which effects the production of these neurotransmitters. When oestrogen levels are higher their productions increases, also extreme fatigue, sleep disorders, depression and anxiety and hot flushes put the body under stress making it difficult to focus. While this may be a major factor in poor concentration factors such as normal aging, poor nutrition, neurological disorders, hyperactivity and drug use may also influence concentration. Memory lapses can also be caused by lack of sleep, excess workload, medication and excessive alcohol consumption. If you experience severe memory lapses (forgetting information you have known for years and use routinely) please consult a doctor. Other illnesses associated with memory lapses include Alzheimer, head trauma, cancer, ADD, stroke, multi-infarct dementia and brain infections (encephalitis or meningitis).

What can I do to prevent these problems?

Try cutting back on alcohol, caffeine and sugar. Eating a healthy diet that is high in nutrients like Omega 3 and 6 (found in fish,

Walnuts and proteins) can help. Keeping stress levels to a minimum will also help. Meditation and yoga can help with this. Also try to do brain activities such as sudoku or crossword puzzles. Intense aerobic exercises can have the same increase on the brains concentration ability as pharmaceutical stimulants such as Ritalin according to 34menopausalsymptoms website. Clearly intense activity is not something most ME sufferers are capable of but any exercise is better than none.

ME sufferers

Here are some of the responses I received relating to the effects of the menopause on their cognitive abilities.

"... foggy brain, lack of concentration"

"... talking to adults is exhausting due to cognitive issues"

" ... (I think) my information processing capability has dropped significantly."

"... even reading is difficult"

"... deterioration in cognitive functioning (particularly short term memory)"

"...unable to drive without becoming dangerously fatigued..."

"I feel disorientated and disconnected and need a lot of silence to regain a degree of normalcy"

Many ME/CFS sufferers experience a level of cognitive problems. It rated as the second highest in MEA survey's list of reported symptoms. Poor concentration and memory and the dreaded brain fog are something that appears to go hand in hand with extreme fatigue. I usually find that it is one of the first signs that tell me I need to rest. It can be extremely frustrating to be unable to say what you mean, or follow a conversation properly. I will often find I am reading a book and am unable to make sense of it, I know the words, I know what they mean but as I read them from the page I am unable to make any sense of it at all. That is when I know I have to rest.

Volunteers reported having difficulty remembering names and finding talking draining. Only 25% listed this as a memory/cognitive problems symptom of the menopause. Others stated that their levels of stamina to complete any task (mental as well as physical) had dropped significantly.

25% of women also reported headaches/migraines that had become worse since entering the menopause.

While some may experience problems others have not noticed any change so you may not notice any difference. If you do experience a migraine it can disturb your vision and make you feel nauseous. Lying in a quiet dark room may help.

Migraines can be extremely debilitating to someone with ME/CFS as it is yet more exhaustion added onto an already exhausted body, therefore it is worth discussing them with your doctor who may be able to help with medication. It is a good idea to keep a diary to try and identify any triggers in your diet or environment so you can eliminate them as much as possible.

What is a migraine?

A migraine is a severe headache with a throbbing pain at the front or one side of the head which affects about 15% of adults in the UK. 1 in 4 of these affected are women and 1 in 12 men. This is believed (although not proven) to be due to fluctuating hormone levels as some women find their migraine attacks are worse around the time of their periods. Some people experience sensitivity to light and nausea. Other symptoms can include sensitivity to sound and smells, nausea, vomiting, poor concentration, sweating, feeling hot or cold, a frequent need to urinate and abdominal pain (sometimes followed by diarrhoea). A migraine can last anywhere from 3 hours to 4 days. You may feel tired for up to 7 days afterwards.

Ocular migraines or migraine with aura may not include a headache but are vision problems related to changes in the blood flow to brain. Symptoms can include flashing lights, disturbed vision and blind spots. The best course of action is to take a mild pain relief to stop a headache following the ocular migraine. Also to sit in a dark room or if not possible try sitting with your eyes shut for at least 10 minutes. Dark glasses may help. Ocular migraines are caused by triggers which can include certain foods, hormonal changes, bright lights or certain medications and can last for up to an hour. They may or may not be followed by a headache. You may experience poor co-ordination and a stiffness or pins and needles. These symptoms usually start 15 minutes to an hour before a headache (which may or may not occur).

Treatments

The best over the counter medication for migraines are 900mg aspirin or 1000mg of paracetamol every four hours. It is best to take this as soon as the headache begins and soluble tablets are absorbed more quickly than solid tablets. Aspirin, strictly speaking, is an anti-inflammatory painkiller, another is ibuprofen. Some brands are dissolvable which can make swallowing them easier especially if you are feeling sick. There are other types of anti-inflammatory painkillers that are available on prescription and all of these should be taken with some food or milk to avoid upsetting your stomach. Always read the list of cautions and side-effects as some people with high blood pressure, asthma, heart or kidney failure may not be able to take anti-inflammatory painkillers.

It is best not to use codeine or medication containing codeine, such as co-codamol, as these can make the migraine worse due to its side-effects which can make nausea and vomiting worse.

Also try to lie in a quiet, dark room especially if you are experiencing any sensitivity to light.

Depression and Anxiety

Depression is common during the menopause. Depression is different to sadness or unhappiness. It is normal to experience sadness or feeling unhappy at setbacks and problems in everyday life. Depression is more severe and lasts for much longer. It is usually accompanied by problems with sleeping and eating disorders, a loss of interest in usual activities and withdrawal from those close to you. Physically you may experience a decrease in energy, fatigue, either overeating or a loss of appetite, excessive sleeping or insomnia yet waking early in the morning. Headaches, problems with cramps or digestions (that do not ease with treatment) and persistent aches and pains are also symptoms. Emotional symptoms include restlessness, irritability, feeling worthless, guilty or helpless, feelings of pessimism or hopelessness, feeling anxious, sad or empty. Behavioural symptoms are finding it difficult to concentrate or make decisions, remembering details and a lack of interest in your usual activities including neglecting your responsibilities and your appearance. To diagnose depression there must have been a persistent feeling of sadness or loss of interest or pleasure for at least two weeks. There must be four other symptoms as well as this feeling for a minimum of two weeks. Major depression can seriously impair your life and your ability to function.

Dystymic disorder usually lasts for more than two years but is less intense than major depression. Adjustment disorder is usually brought on by a stressful situation or event and last for less than six months. If it lasts longer it is described as acute or chronic. Seasonal affective Disorder (SAD) is depression that is caused by lack of sunlight in the winter month. Manic depression or Bipolar disorder can be very severe. Symptoms are unusual shifts in energy and moods, and limit the ability to function which is caused by this brain disorder. Psychotic depression has delusions and psychosis as symptoms and sufferers may have hallucinations or irrational thoughts and fears.

Anxiety can be as slight as mild agitation right through to physical symptoms such as pain attacks, rapid heartbeats, shortness of breath and palpitations. Both depression and anxiety are serious symptoms of the menopause which can be extremely disruptive to your quality of life. Women between the ages of 45-55 are four times more likely to experience depression than those younger.

If untreated, depression can lead to a greater risk of osteoporosis and heart attacks.

Panic attacks happen when you become so anxious that you begin to hyperventilate. You may feel as if you are having a heart attack because of the tightness in your chest. Other symptoms are a pounding heartbeat, sweating, feeling faint, nausea, shaky limbs, and legs turning to jelly, discomfort breathing, chest pains and fear of losing control. It can be very frightening and over whelming. You may feel as if you are blacking out or even going mad. Symptoms occur very quickly and are an exaggeration of the body's normal response to fear, excitement or stress. They usually last between 5 and 20 minutes, peaking with 10 minutes. Some people experience one attack after another or are so anxious afterward that they think they are lasting longer. The frequency of having another attack can vary drastically from person to person with some having them several times a week, once a month, having one or two and never have another one. They can come without any warning and appear random. They can even come on during the night and wake you up. In America around 6 million adults suffer from panic disorders with it affecting twice as many women as men.

What causes this?

Depression and anxiety can be caused by hormone imbalances. Oestrogen is important in helping regulate the functions of the brain. This includes the chemicals serotonin and cortisol which influences moods. The decreasing oestrogen also causes physical and mental symptoms which in turn can lead to depression. Personality, disease, your environment and genetics can also cause depression as can biochemical factors.

Panic attacks can be brought on by experiencing traumatic events (Post Traumatic Stress Disorder), fears/phobias, and Obsessive Compulsive Disorder (OCD).

Treatments

Depression and anxiety are not something to be taken lightly and you should always be guided by your doctor. There are a wide variety of prescription drugs which can help you cope more effectively. There are however some ways in which you can help yourself. A healthy diet can help to stabilize moods. Practicing relaxation such as mediation or yoga can help alleviate anxiety. There are several therapies such as acupuncture, massage, aromatherapy, bio feed and hypnosis which can help. Exercise such as walking, jogging, cycling or swimming for 30 minutes three times a week can also help alleviate symptoms. Try to sleep for 7-8 hours a day and stay hydrated. Vitamins B, C, D and E as well as a healthy diet are also said to help. Try to avoid alcohol and caffeine. Alcohol is a temporary fix which while seeming to help actually leads to deeper depression as well as possible vitamin deficiency. Depression can make you crave sugary things and both they and coffee will give an energy boost until they wear off, then they will leave you feeling down and anxious. Try to eat a diet rich in foods that promote oestrogen production such as soy, apples, alfalfa, cherries, rice, wheat, potatoes and yams.

There are also herbal supplements available which I have covered in the alternative medicine section.

You can learn to control panic attacks using breathing and relaxation techniques, assertiveness training can help to feel more confident (and therefore more relaxed) and complimentary therapies can also be beneficial. Talking therapies and learning to face up to your problems. Therapies such as CBT (Cognitive Behavioural Therapy) can be useful. This will usually involve 6-12 hourly sessions (once a week). Medication is another alternative. This can be in the form of anti-depressants, beta-blockers, tranquillizers and sleeping pills which may relieve symptoms but will not get to the cause of it.

How does it affect those with ME/CFS?

Depression is often a side effect of chronic illness. We grieve for the loss of our old life and the future may seem bleak. Our loss of independence and our "old life" can be devastating. We feel that we are losing control over our lives. Chronic pain can make us irritable and difficult to live with. It can also intensify feelings of helplessness and hopelessness. When there seems little to look forward to except a lifetime filled with limitations and pain it is easy to become down and depressed. Unfortunately this appears to increase our sensitivity to yet more pain. Biologically depression and chronic pain share some of the same neurotransmitters and nerve pathways. If you used exercise and activities as a coping method you are now denied this as an option. Chronic pain and depression are often treated together because they are intertwined, one affecting the other.

Anti-depressants are often used to treat both pain and depression because they use many of the same neurotransmitters. They work on the brain to reduce the perception of pain. Tricyclic antidepressants (e.g. Elavin and doxepin) have been shown to be effective but because of their side-effects their use is limited. Newer antidepressants such as Cymbalta and Effexor which are known as serotonin and norepinephrine reuptake inhibitors seems to work well with less side effects.

St John's Wort is a popular herbal remedy used to combat depression. It is available in tablet form and is also available in oil form. Care must be taken if being used as oil (although oil form is usually used to treat bruises, wounds and muscle pain and not depression) as it can cause serious sensitivity to sunlight. It can also interfere with other medications which can be dangerous. It is best to have a break between coming off prescribed medication and beginning to take this and please always obtain advice from a qualified source before making any decisions regarding medication at all.

Cognitive therapies can help where patients learn to recognize negative thoughts and to realize that these are often a distortion of reality. A patient can then learn to change their reactions and thought patterns which will improve their experiences of pain.

The MEA survey actually showed that the effectiveness of both St John's Wort and CBT scored higher than tradition medication in sufferer's opinions. It shows that a combination of the two may be an effective way to deal with depression.

Of those who contacted me, many reported symptoms ranging from mood swings to anxiety and depression. 72% of women responded yes when asked if they suffered from depression or mood swings against 27% saying no. This was broken down as.

9%	reporting mood swings
9%	reporting this settling after their periods stopped
18%	reported their condition being stabilized by medication
27%	reported this as only since the menopause or condition worsening after the menopause.
9%	yes

If you suspect you are suffering from depression then you should consult your doctor who will recommend the appropriate course of action for you.

Mood swings

This can include feelings of irritability or aggression. It also includes frequent mood changes especially depression and sadness, feeling nervous and anxious and experiencing increased stress levels. You may lack any motivation or feel tearful or unexplainably emotional. Up to 75% of women suffer from mood swing when going though the menopause. If you have experienced post partum (post natal) depression or PMS you are more likely to experience mood swings during the menopause. The MEA survey showed that more than half those taking part experienced some level of mood swings.

What causes this?

This is mainly caused by changes in hormones, particular the effect of oestrogen levels on the production of serotonin as it is a mood regulating neurotransmitter.

Treatments

Balancing hormone levels will help with this. There is a range of supplements that can help. See the chapter on Alternative Therapies. HRT may also help by restoring your hormone levels.

Fatigue

This is something anyone who has ME/CFS is already familiar with. Fatigue is described as a sudden overwhelming weakness, exhaustion and reduced energy level. There is a difference between Chronic Fatigue Syndrome and fatigue associated with the menopause. The physical symptoms of menopausal fatigue are fatigue after eating, crashing fatigue, muscle fatigue and drowsiness. The mental symptoms are decreased wakefulness and attention, apathy, irritability, memory lapse and trouble concentrating.

The fatigue experienced from ME also includes extreme fatigue after physical and mental exertion that is disproportional to that of someone without the condition. Typically sufferers also experience a slower recovery from fatigue.

What causes it?

It is caused by temporary hormone imbalances made worse by lack of sleep, stress, irritability. It affects up to 80% of menopausal women.

What can I do?

HRT can help to balance out your hormones. Other approaches include lifestyle changes such as reducing your stress levels (try yoga or meditation) and trying to get a good night's sleep (cutting out alcohol and caffeine may help). Diet, you can try eating more alkaline forming foods (leafy greens, almonds, beets, figs, parsley and dates) as these have been shown to boost ph levels in the blood and boost energy levels. Alternative medicine – many women try aromatherapy, massage, acupuncture and bio-feeds. Herbal supplements are another option to treat a hormone imbalance. There are two types of herbs that are used to treat fatigue. These are phytoestrogenic herbs like Black Cohosh containing estrogenic components produced by plants. They treat the imbalance initially by introducing plants based estrogens into the body (but the result of adding outside hormones means the woman's body may become less capable of producing oestrogen on its own, further decreasing the body's own hormone level) and non-estrogenic herbs which do not contain oestrogen. These nourish the pituitary and endocrine glands, stimulating them to produce natural hormones efficiently, balancing the oestrogen levels. They help the body create its own hormones and are considered the safest way to treat menopausal symptoms (e.g. Macafem)

"MACAFEM nutrients help restore natural hormones in women. Unlike hormone drugs, which are basically resumed in taking synthetic hormones, Macafem acts totally differently in your body. It nourishes and stimulates your own natural hormone production, by inducing the optimal functioning of the pituitary and endocrine glands"

Quote from Nature and Health magazine (Dr Chacon)

How does it affects ME sufferers?

As anyone who suffers from ME/CFS will know fatigue is one of the main features of the illness and as it is listed as a symptom of the menopause I was concerned about any increase in the level of fatigue I should expect. The responses I received from women broke down as follows

53% Reported experiencing more severe fatigue

29% Reported fatigue levels stayed the same, (12% started the menopause at the same time so were unable to distinguish between the two).

18% Reported fatigue had or was improving, (6% got worse but then improved- these are also include in the 53% as well)

While this confirms that the menopause may have a negative effect on your fatigue levels it also shows that it isn't a certainty. Hot flushes and night sweats were stated as a major reason for increased fatigue. This was partly due to disturbed sleep. Stamina also seemed to have reduced in some women. On the plus side those that reported improvement said that the absence of periods meant that their levels of fatigue had improved and that the fluctuation of symptoms had become less than before the menopause.

I haven't included my own response to this question in the statistics as it seems to vary from week to week. At times I feel much more tired but I have also had times where I felt better than I have in the last 15 years.

Pacing and managing you energy levels are crucial to minimizing fatigue levels.

"The worst thing I feel is aching and weakness in my legs which comes in phases and seems to be linked to my menopause hormone levels e.g. if I'm having a bad flushes time then I generally have weak fatigued legs and generally feel unwell."

"(fatigue levels) have become more severe and I am tired by 5 or 6pm and find concentrating on conversation very tiring."

"I find I get tired more quickly now"

Hot flushes or hot flashes

Referred to as either flushes or flashes this is an intense sudden hot feeling in the upper body and face. It may by accompanied, or proceeded, by sweating, rapid heartbeat, nausea, dizziness, headache, weakness and anxiety. You may be left sweating and reddened. It may last from a few seconds to several minutes but occasionally up to an hour and can take up to half an hour to feel ok afterwards.

There are two types of flushes. The standard flush comes on quickly reaching intensity in as little as a minute and lasting a few minutes before subsiding. The second is referred to as a slow hot flush or ember flushes. This appears as quickly as a standard one but lasts for around half an hour. A woman may continue to get ember flushes after her standard hot flushes have stopped.

The most common time for a woman to get a hot flush is 6-8am and 6-9pm.

For younger women or women who have experienced a surgical menopause (i.e. a hysterectomy) hot flushes are generally more intense than in older women and may continue until the natural age of the menopause.

What causes them?

They are mainly caused by hormonal changes although they can be triggered by medication and lifestyle. When the hypothalamus (the part of the brain responsible for controlling appetite, sleep cycle, sex hormones and body temperature) experiences a drop in oestrogen it gets confused and makes you "too hot". It is not sure how this drop confuses the hypothalamus but it thinks you are overheating and results in the brain trying to get rid of this heat from the body. To do this it makes your heart pump faster, dilating the blood vessels in the skin to circulate the blood, activating you sweat glands to cool you down. Some women's skin temperature can rise by up to 6 degrees at these times. It is reported that up to 85% of women experience hot flushes during the approach to and the first few years after their periods stop. 20% experience severe problems with hot flushes. The average time affected by them is 2 years although 10% can experience them for over 15 years, 20-50% of these women continue to experience them for years afterwards although the intensity decreases with time.

What can I do about them?

There are several approaches which can help alleviate this symptom. As they are caused by fluctuating hormone levels you can try to correct this imbalance. You can also make some changes to your lifestyle which may help.

On a day to day basis you should look for things that may be triggering an attack. Common ones are alcohol, caffeine, spicy foods, hot foods, hot tubs, saunas, hot showers, hot room/beds, hot weather and smoking. If you find these trigger an attack try to avoid them for a while and keep a diary to pin down what affects you.

Dress in layers so you can take clothes off quickly if you start to feel hot. Choosing cottons, linens and rayon is better than wool, synthetics or silk. You may find that open necked shirts are more comfortable than turtlenecks or polo-necked jumpers. Cotton sheets and nightwear are also advisable. If you have room and can afford, consider a larger bed so you have plenty of space and are not touching your partner when having a flush. Don't rush before bed, try to be calm and if possible take a cool shower. Have a hand held fan and a cool drink next to the bed at night so you can cool down without getting up immediately. Try to keep the bedroom cool. Recommended temperatures seem to vary from 18.3-22.2 degrees Celsius (65-72 degrees Fahrenheit). Warmer rooms can raise the core body temperature which increases the likelihood of hot flushes. www.SleepBetter.org suggests you use products which help provide relief from night sweats and hot flushes. In particular they suggest Carpenter Co's Isotonic (R), Iso-cool (TM) pillows and mattress toppers which both help adjust to the body's changing body temperature by absorbing heat to regulate body warmth and create a cooling sensation to provide a better night's sleep. They also feature a science based personal sleep profile which will give a guide to getting a better night's sleep based on you as an individual.

Try sipping iced water to take your temperature down. Also turn your heating down (you can save money on your heating bills too!) and perhaps invest in a fan or air-conditioning.

According to an article in the Daily Mail (25/11/12) by Anna Hodgekiss a study carried out by the University of Taylor and Baylor University in the US have shown that hypnotherapy can have a beneficial effect on reducing hot flushes. It showed an 80% decrease in the frequency and severity of hot flushes in the group of women receiving hypnotherapy treatment compared to a 15% decrease in those women who simply met and discussed their symptoms with their doctor. Also the skin temperature monitors showed a 57% decrease in comparison with 10% of the control group. As a hypnotherapist I have had a reduction in the frequency and intensity of my hot flushes and my general overall health when I regularly practice hypnotherapy on myself.

ME sufferers and hot flushes

The MEA survey reported that 63% listed "inability to cope with temperature change (night sweats)" as a major problem and 28% as a minor problems. Clearly this is a problem for ME sufferers before we even consider the hormonal changes which occur causing hot flushes during the menopause. Obviously some of these women may have also been going through the menopause and, as I have found, it can be difficult to identify whether it is an ME night sweat or a menopausal one. From the responses I received hot flushes were top of the worse symptoms of the menopause, often accompanied by headaches, disturbed sleep and overall weakness/reduced stamina levels. Problems sleeping and the excess fatigue were attributed to the hot flushes so if you can do anything to reduce their frequency or severity then it will be beneficial.

"HRT and cutting out sugar has helped stop the horrible night sweats."

"They are not so bad they affect my energy levels, they are just uncomfortable and inconvenient and mean I have to change my clothes more often"

"The hot flushes were the worst. I did try taking some soya based alternative tablets which helped somewhat."

"If I have a bad session with flushes it seems to weaken my body even more ... a hot flush suddenly comes on and I feel weak, nauseous and really unwell, even faint unlike other people who do not have ME"

"Hot flushes left me drained and exhausted. All I want to do was lie down and sleep."

Incontinence

There are three main types of incontinence. Firstly, Stress Incontinence, this is where you accidentally urinate if you sneeze, laugh, cough or physically exert yourself. Secondly, Urge Incontinence, this is when the bladder contracts and empties itself despite your efforts to stop it and finally Overflow Incontinence, where you lose the sensation that you have to go and don't know when your bladder is full.

Stress Incontinence – As a woman gets older the pelvic muscles often grow weaker and the walls between the bladder and vagina weaken. This leads to sudden pressure if you laugh sneeze etc which squeezes the bladder and causes leakages.

Urge Incontinence – This is sometimes referred to as an over active, spastic bladder or reflex incontinence.

Overflow Incontinence – Constant or frequent dribbling. Sufferers often only produce a weak flow when going to the toilet and feel that they have never fully emptied their bladder. Diabetes can result in nerve damage which causes this problem.

It is reported that 13million of Americans suffer with incontinence and 85% of these are women. Around 40% of menopausal and postmenopausal suffer from this condition.

What causes this?

Oestrogen not only helps the health of the urinary tract lining as well as keeping a woman's muscles strong. As oestrogen levels drop approaching the menopause and the bladder becomes more difficult to control as the muscles weaken. Other causes of incontinence are weight gain, previous pregnancies (weakened muscles), infections, nerve damage (from stroke or diabetes), heart problems, depression and tranquillizers, medications (particularly diuretics) and difficulty moving.

Treatments

Strengthening the pelvic floor muscles (the muscles that support the bladder) can help. Caffeine and tobacco can lead to a worsening of the condition. Trying to improve your hormonal balance can also help. For prolonged problems please consult your doctor as there are medications that can help alleviate the symptoms but do be aware of side effects.

Pelvic Floor Exercises

This involves strengthening the pelvic floor muscles so that they can then support the bladder more effectively and reduce the problem of incontinence. First you need to be able to identify which muscles need to be strengthened. Initially tighten the muscles around your anus (back passage) as if you are trying to stop passing wind, do not tense any other muscles such as the buttocks or thighs. Next tighten the muscles further forward as if you are trying to stop urination. You should be able to notice a difference. It is those muscles further forward that you need to strengthen. You should do the following exercises for a minimum of 3 months although it may take long for the best improvement. It is a good idea to try and incorporate these exercises into your daily routine and not just until your incontinence has improved. If you tone muscles but then stop exercising they will not maintain that level of strengthen.

- Slowly pull up and tighten the pelvic floor muscles as hard as you can and hold for the count of 5 before releasing. Repeat 5 times

- Tighten the pelvic floor muscles quickly and hold for the count of 2 before releasing. Repeat 5 times
- Continue to alternate these two exercises for 5 minutes.
- Do these exercises at least 3 times a day (although 6-10 times)
- Only squeeze these muscles, do not squeeze the buttocks or thighs
- Remember to keep your knees slightly apart. These exercises can be done sitting, standing or lying down.

If you are having difficulty and need help performing these exercises there are other aids to help you strengthen your pelvic floor muscles which your physiotherapist may suggest.
These are –

Electrical Stimulation – A special electrical device stimulates the pelvic floor muscles aiming to make the contact harder.

Vaginal Cones – Small plastic cones that are inserted into the vagina twice a day for 15 minutes. They come in different weights (you start with the lightest) and progress onto the heavier weights. You need to use your pelvic floor muscles to hold these in place which will strengthen them.

Biofeedback – Your physiotherapist or continence advisor can help ensure you are exercising the correct muscles by inserting an electrical device into the vagina which will make a sound or signal when you are squeezing the correct muscles.

Other devices – There are other devices advertised but any of these should be used in addition to not instead of your basic pelvic floor muscles as there is little research into how these work (most work on the principle of inserting something into the vagina that you are then required to squeeze) so it is best to be guided by your health advisor.

The benefits of doing these exercises even if you do not suffer from incontinence are that you are less likely to encounter problems if your muscles are strong. There is an added benefit in that having strong pelvic floor muscles is report to heighten sexual pleasure for some women.

Osteoporosis

Osteoporosis literally means Porous Bone. It is a thinning and weakening of the bone along with a decrease in bone mass and density. This makes them break or fracture more easily. A third of women over the age of 50 will experience fractures as a result of osteoporosis (according to patient.co.uk it is 50%). It affects women more than men who have stronger, bulkier bones which don't lose mass as easily - 80% of sufferers are women. Patient.co.uk state "by 70 years of age some women will have lost 30% of their bone material". When we are aging our bodies make new bone more slowly than we lose old bone and by the age of 35 there is more bone removal than renewal. Oestrogen helps calcium be absorbed into the bone. The rate at which bone density reduces increases as oestrogen levels drop. There is no pain as this progresses and can go unnoticed until weakened bone cause painful fractures (usually in the back and hips).

What causes this?

During the menopause oestrogen levels drop. The drop in oestrogen and aging are the reason for this condition. Bones are a living tissue made up of collagen fibres (which are tough and elastic) and minerals (which are a hard gritty material) which contain cells that make, mould and reabsorb bone. While you grow you produce bone more quickly than you reabsorb it. This situation changes as you age and you start to lose bone making them weaker and less dense.

Risk factors for bone loss and osteoporosis

- Family history – i.e. parents or siblings have been affected

- A BMI of 19 or below and are very underweight. Illnesses like anorexia nervosa leave oestrogen levels low for long periods of time which combined with a poor diet can affected the bones
- Lack of and vitamin D – a result of poor diet and lack of sunlight
- Premature menopause
- If your periods have stopped for 6 months to a year before menopause (this can be caused by over-exercising and extreme dieting)
- If you smoke
- If you drink more than 4 units of alcohol a day
- If you have had a bone fracture after a bump or minor fall already
- If you have lead a particularly sedentary lifestyle (especially during your teenage years) or have never taken any exercise
- Steroid medication – a side effect of steroid medication is bone loss (usually if prescribed for 3 months or more). Conditions such as Arthritis and Asthma are sometimes controlled by long-term courses of steroids
- Certain medical conditions can affect your bones i.e. overactive thyroid, chronic liver disease, Cushing's syndrome, Crohn's disease, rheumatoid arthritis, chronic kidney failure, type 1 diabetes or any condition that causes poor mobility

Prevention

Exercise and Lifestyle

Exercise will improve the strength of your bones as well as reduce the risk of heart disease, high blood pressure and diabetes. Exercises that are beneficial for preventing osteoporosis are weight bearing ones such as walking and aerobics.

Stopping Smoking

Women who smoke tend to experience an earlier menopause and often produce less oestrogen which can lead to increased bone loss. Fractures take longer to heal in smokers than non-smokers. Smokers with a broken leg take 62% longer to heal than non-smokers.

Diet

It is essential to have a good calcium intake throughout your life to have healthy bones. A healthy intake of calcium for adults is approx 800mg.

Good sources of calcium are dairy products, white bread and calcium fortified soya milk. Low and higher fat dairy products contain the same amounts of calcium. Cow's milk contains 300mg of calcium per 250ml (half a pint), so does 150g (5oz) of yogurt.

If your diet is low in calcium supplements can be taken. Vitamin D is needed for the absorption of calcium, therefore if you have poor mobility and are frail and elderly a calcium supplement with vitamin D may help but do discuss this with your doctor.

Treatments (Most common)

HRT

This reduces the rate of bone loss by replacing the oestrogen. It is beneficial if it is started early in the menopause and is taken for at least 5 years. You should always discuss the risks of HRT with your doctor before deciding if the benefits outweigh the risks to you and your personal medical situation. (See chapter on HRT)

Bisphosphates

Alendronic Acid (Fosamax) and **Disodium Etidronate (Didronel PMO)** are two commonly used. These help with bone strength overtime by slowing the rate at which bone is dissolved. It is often used (for men and women) when using steroid drugs.

Risedronate Sodium (Actonel) and **Ibandronic Acid (Bonviva)** are similar but are only used in women after the menopause.

Alendronic acid and Risendronate Sodium reduces fractures of the spine and hip while Etidronate and Bandronic Acid have only been shown to reduce spine fractures.

There are side-effects including abdominal pain, diarrhoea, constipation and indigestion with these and each has to be taken differently. Due to the irritation and ulceration of the oesophagus they have strict instruction on how to be taken.

Strontium Ranelate (Protelos)

This is used in postmenopausal women who can't take bisphospanates.

It has been shown to increase the formation of bone in addition to decreasing the breakdown of bone, therefore reducing hip and spinal fractures.

Raloxifen (Evista)

This is used in postmenopausal woman to prevent and treat osteoporosis. This medicine is called a selective oestrogen receptor modulation (SERM).

This has an anti-oestrogen effect on breast tissue and the womb (uterus) while stimulating bone growth in the way oestrogens do.

This can make it a desirable alternative to using HRT (which has as increased risk of breast cancer) but it may increase the risk of blood clots in the veins. It carries similar risks to HRT regarding thrombosis and can't be used by women with a history of DVT (deep vein thrombosis). It has been shown to reduce spinal fractures but not hip fractures and is preferably only used in women who are past the menopause by 5 years.

ME Sufferers

The main issue here is the restrictions that ME/CFS put on exercise. When getting dressed seems like a monumental achievement then the idea of any exercise seems impossible. This would appear to make women with ME/CFS more susceptible to osteoporosis and increased bone loss. Some exercise is going to be better than none. I have listed some types of exercise that may be possible for sufferers under the Chapter Exercise. Therefore it is simply a case of doing what you can, ensuring that your diet is rich in calcium and taking supplements if required.

Also ME sufferers are less likely to spend time outside therefore restricting the amount of sunlight their bodies receive. As vitamin D is essential in the absorption of calcium either investigate taking a supplement and try to spend some time outside in the sunlight to ensure your body has the levels it needs.

Stopping smoking and keeping alcohol to below 4 units may not be a problem as many people with ME find that they cannot tolerate alcohol and are sensitive to pollutants such as cigarette smoke. It is believed that women ME/CFS sufferers are at a high risk of developing osteoporosis, especially in the time around the menopause. Research by the Royal North Shore Hospital in Sydney Australia backs this up.

Pain

This can include headaches, breast and joint pain. Headaches may be worse in the early stages of the menopause. Breast pain is common before or with period pains but also in pregnancy, breast feeding and the menopause. This can be painful to touch and include tenderness, soreness, swelling, burning and tightness. It can affect one or both breast and can be constant or intermittent. Joint pain associated with the menopause and includes pain, swelling, warmth and stiffness in the joints. It is common for women experiencing joint pain to feel stiffness in the morning (limiting movement) which is made worse with exercise.

What causes this?

Headaches can be caused by a drop in your oestrogen levels, although common illnesses (like the flu), muscle tension and drinking too much alcohol can also contribute to them. If they are severe please consult your doctors.

Breast pain is the result of hormonal changes. The medical name for this is Mastalgia, Mastodynia and Mammalgia. If you have any lumps, discharge or changes (such as colour) please consult your doctor. Other less common reasons for pain are trauma, cysts, medication (antidepressants, oral contraception, HRT, cholesterol and heart drugs), stress, alcoholism, previous surgery, breast size or mastitis.

Doctors are not sure why but oestrogen keeps the inflammation in joints down. Therefore as the oestrogen levels drop inflammation increases and results in joint pain.

Treatments

The best option is to try and balance your hormones. This includes lifestyle changes and avoiding dietary triggers which can help. Natural therapies may help you target the hormonal imbalance in the body. Pain can be relieved by resting. Other non hormonal related causes are wear and tear, weight and diet, muscle loss, no exercise, injuries, stress, hereditary, bone disease and metabolic disorders, tumours, cancer and inflammation of the joints. Do consult a doctor if the pain is accompanied by fever, weight loss accompanied with joint pain, if it worsens and moves to other joints and lasts for more than 3 days. If you are concerned please discuss this with your doctors.

Pain, ME and the menopause

Up to 75% of ME/CFS sufferers are affected by muscle pain.

Aspirin – this is an anti-inflammatory drug which can be helpful although it is advised that you take it with food to minimize stomach irritation. Prolonged use can leading to bleeding of the stomach lining. Some have a slow onset of action which means they can be useful at night.

Paracetamol – Less effective than aspirin in controlling muscle and joint pain as it has little anti-inflammatory action. You should not take more than the recommend dose of 8 x 500g in 24 hours (or this quantity for a prolong time) as some people can be extremely sensitive to even low doses.

The MEA survey showed that aspirin and paracetamol produced the fewest adverse effects whilst having a positive effect for 48% of sufferers.

Codeine – This is sometimes combined with aspirin or

paracetamol which can be used for mild to moderate pain relief. Common combinations are Co-Codamol and Co-Codaprin. Long-term use can cause constipation as well as dizziness, nausea and sedation.

Caffeine is best avoided as it may aggravate gastric problems.

Tramadol – is a stronger form of analgesic which is between codeine and morphine. A short course of this pain relief has been shown to be useful to ME sufferers. The MEA survey reported this as the drug which helped best with pain (which as this is prescribed for severe or terminal pain is not surprising) for 63% of those completing the survey they also noted that the benefits of taking it should be carefully weighed against the significant dangers of taking opiate (morphine based) drugs. Whether it is ideal for this type of painkiller to be used on a general basis is debatable.

NSAIDs (Non-steroidal anti-inflammatory drugs) are a mild analgesic that may help with muscle and joint pain as well as headache. Ibuprofen (sold as brufen) and is available over the counter or on prescription and it does have side-effects including stomach irritation, blood problems, bleeding and rashes (therefore care must be taken if you have any history of stomach ulcers). These drugs were reported to be beneficial for 53% for sufferers in the MEA survey.

Other drugs – Low doses of sedating tricyclic anti-depressants can help improve sleep and relieve mild pain throughout the body. Examples of these are Adapin, Sibeguan (Doxepin), Elavil, Etafon, Libitrol, Triavil (Amitriptyline), Norepramin (Desipramine), Pamelor (Nortriptylin).

SSRI/SNRI anti-depressants (Selective Serotonin Reuptake

Inhibitors or Serotonin norepinephrine Reuptake Inhibitors) help because serotonin helps with your sleep-wake cycle as well as processing pain and norepinephrine is involved in stress response and energy bursts. Examples of these are Cymbalta (Duloxetine), Prozac (fluoxetine), Zoloft (Sertraline), Paxil (Paroxetine), Effexor (Venlafaxine), Desvrel (Trazodone) and Wellbutrin (Bupropion).

You may be able to ease pain to some degree with warm baths or a hot water bottle. For localized pain treatments such as Deep Heat may provide some relief. Alternative therapies may help. Massages can help ease pain caused by tension as can relaxation although it should be gentle especially if the muscles are tender. Hypnotherapy and talking therapies can help you to manage your pain effectively as well as reduce stress and tension which may help. Acupuncture has been shown to help with pain relief with 48% of sufferers reporting it had a good to moderate effect on their pain levels. Please see the chapter on Alternative Therapies.

"Sometimes the floor would feel as though it was coming up to hit me and I would frequently wake up with a sore throat and pain in my arms and legs just like when the glandular fever began."

"It's not just pain but the whole host of ME symptoms that appear after a day filled with hot flushes"

"...because I am having some periods when I am exhausted all my muscles feel sore and tender..."

"All my ME symptoms are exaggerated including pain in my muscles and joints especially on waking up"

"Sometimes the pain in my muscles and joints is so intense I can't sleep and have to take additional painkillers. This hasn't changed

much with the menopause because it always happened when I had a period but does happen more at times when I am feeling very tired or I have other menopausal symptoms."

"My stamina has dropped and I find I tire more easily. My ME symptoms, including pain, seems to come on much more quickly now I am going through the menopause."

Sex, the menopause and ME

The one thing that is obvious from the response I received is that many women feel guilty about their 'lack of' sex lives. On top of an illness that can rob us of the ability to live a 'normal' life, women are experiencing guilt about their feelings towards sex. They might have been rejecting their husbands and partners because they have felt tired and uncomfortable due to their CFS/ME but now this can be made worse as the menopause takes its toll and their desire decreases as well.

Sex is a subject that isn't often talked when discussing illness. A lack of energy, pain and sometimes a lack of self-confidence that often comes from your life changing can all make it something that we try to ignore. It is important to remember that sex is a normal and natural activity. It is an intimate act which lays us bare, if you'll pardon the pun, so many people are reluctant to talk about it.

According to Robert Rothrock of Pain Concern 75% of chronic pain sufferers experience some form of sexual dysfunction and he advises that people should resume sexual activity as soon as possible after an illness.

Libido

A lack of libido can have a huge effect on a relationship. It is one thing to have your sex life curtailed by pain or lack of energy but no longer desiring your partner is bound to put a strain on any relationship. I was surprised at the number of women who reported to not having had sex for over a year. They often stated that their low libido had dwindled to none. Good communication is always a positive step but it is important not to choose a time when you are extremely emotional. It might seem obvious but trying to explain how you feel to your partner through floods of tears or while you are snarling like a rabid dog is not going to be productive.

The responses to this part of the questionnaire have been limited. This has partly been because those who did complete this section had other medical problems which either prevented or limited their sex lives. Also some volunteers do not have partners at all so did not complete that section. Those that did were very frank and open with their responses.

Has the menopause affected how often you have sex?

60%   they had less sex (50% of these now don't have sex at all or haven't had for over a year, although 10% did not have a partner at this time)
30%   do not have sex (20% because of either their or their partner's illness)
10%   have more sex

Do you reject your partner?
14%   No
86%   Yes

Do you feel guilty about the lack of sex in your relationship?
25%   No
75%   Yes

Is sex more painful since the onset of the menopause?
14%   No
86%   Yes

Do you feel your partner understands the changes you are going through?

78%   Yes (55% said only partially or they "thought" so)

22%   No

Has it created emotional distance and do you think you partner feels rejected?

37.5% Yes or sometimes

62.5% No

Although most information on the menopause suggests a decline in libido is normal there are a growing number of articles about woman who are saying the complete opposite. As with ME and CFS it seems that each individual is different. Just because libido may decline or decrease during the menopause this is not necessarily a permanent state. On a positive note there were some responses that indicated an increase in libido stating that their sex lives had improved dramatically. At the risk of repeating myself, clearly everybody is different and it is not a case that you will definitely experience a drop in libido.

It is possible that a lack of libido can be due to women adjusting to the end of their reproductive lives and because they feel anxious about the body changes they face as they grow older. Grey hairs, wrinkles, possible weight gain can all contribute to poor body image. Add in the pressures of aging parents and changes in the family dynamic such as children leaving home, it is understandable that some women may feel anxious and uneasy about the future. Changes can make us feel inadequate. Talking about these feelings can help you start to feel better about yourself. Making positive changes such as tackling any weight issues can help with your body image. After all we have to start liking ourselves before we believe that someone else can.

It may be that medication is also affecting your libido. Anti-depressants, tranquillizers, sedatives and narcotic pain medication can decrease sexual desire. So can antihistamines and some blood pressure and heart medication (men can also have difficulty obtaining and maintaining an erection). People who used alcohol or marijuana (cannabis) to self-medicate can also experience a decreased libido (and impotency).

For many couples a dwindling libido may not be an issue but just another change to adjust to. This can become a gentler more peaceful lifestyle where an active sex life is not something that is missed. It is important to remember that a reduction in sexual desire and an active sex life are not a problem unless you find it distressing. You and your partner may simply find that this is all part of your relationship maturing and that less sex is not necessarily something that needs to be fixed. You can still have a loving, intimate relationship without sex if that is what you both want. Communication is important as both partners might feel guilty about their lack of libido unnecessarily. You have to decide what is right for you as a couple as well as you as an individual. After all, it is your relationship and it is individual to you as a couple, so if lack of sex isn't a problem, stop worrying about it.

Check that you are not suffering from a low level of depression. If you are already taking anti-depressants check with your doctor as these can affect libido. It may be beneficial to discuss changing medication with your doctor. Ask for a blood test for low thyroid function and iron deficiency anaemia as both of these affect the sex drive. A lack of libido can be helped by HRT which replaces the lost hormones. Whilst Ginkgo Biloba, Dong Quai, Black Cohosh and Horny Goat Weed are also said to have the same effect by balancing hormones, improving blood flow and raising mood and energy levels and alleviating vaginal dryness. Sexual arousal in women is highly linked to psychological and emotional factors so remember that it is natural for how you are feeling to affect your sex life.

Sex may become painful for some women. This is usually because of vaginal dryness although some experience pain during sex. Some women do experience more difficulty becoming aroused and less sensation around the genitals along with more frequent bladder and bowel infections. If you add in a lower libido and it all sounds rather bleak but do remember that although half of women will experience one of these symptoms there are many who experience none. Therefore please don't expect that you will experience all of them.

Putting sex back on the agenda

It is easy to become fearful of pain during sex if you are in chronic pain or are worried that sex will make the pain worse. If you want sex to be part of your life then you need to start planning for it. Firstly you will need to budget it to fit in around your energy levels. Sex when you are exhausted already is not going to be appealing. Choose a time when your energy levels are at their highest, also choose a time when your pain medication is at its best and your pain levels are at their lowest. Spontaneous sex can be great but so can planned sex. Sex is not just something to save for before you go to sleep especially as night-time can be one of the worse times for people in chronic pain.

Here are some basic tips

- Know your best time
- Take a warm bath or shower and ask your partner to gently massage are sore muscles or joints
- Make sure the bed is warm (an electric blanket may help)

- Choose positions that are comfortable
- Speak to your partner. They are not mind-readers. If you are uncomfortable or in pain then tell them
- Remember you can be intimate without intercourse

On a positive note to quote Robert Rothrock "You may be surprised to learn that research shows that sexual activity when comfortable is often followed by several hours of pain relief!"

Also "The illustrated guide to better sex for people with chronic pain by Robert W Rothrock & Gabriella D'Amore" is worth reading.

Dryness

Lubrications such as K-Y Jelly can be used to help with this but not petroleum based jelly as it can harbour bacteria which can lead to infections

Prescription testosterone creams and gels can be applied to the vagina or clitoris area to increase orgasms and increase sensation.

Localized oestrogen therapy places oestrogen directly into the vagina making sex more comfortable by soothing vaginal tissue and allowing the necessary secretion. These are available as vaginal peccaries, creams or rings which sit inside the vagina and overtime give off small doses of hormones. Unlike oral oestrogens which carry some cancer risks these are generally considered to be safe.

Vitamin E, if applied several times a week, is said to rehydrate vagina tissue. It can be bought in capsule form and if split the contents can be applied. Lubricants containing vitamin E can also be used which can help with problems such as dryness and associated pain during intercourse and possibly even increase sensation. These can be bought without a prescription.

<u>**TIPS**</u>

- Try to maintain some levels of intimacy
- Keep communicating with your partner
- HRT may help with decreasing libido
- Do not be embarrassed about discussing this with your doctor
- Try taking Evening Primrose Oil

In your own words

"My interest in sex did decline (although not disappear). I also increasingly suffered with pain on intercourse, which didn't help. I haven't had a partner for some years and to be honest I don't feel I have the energy to deal with one. The hormonally produced decline in libido means I'm far less inclined to look for one."

"The lack of pain and bloating make relationships easier and I want to be intimate more often."

"...our sex life is now non-existent as I am too tired in the evenings and the after effects are not worth it. My libido is very low so I don't really miss sex (which we don't have any more). Now you highlight it, it is since the menopause symptoms started as I would find time in the best part of my day before."

"Lack of libido with ME fatigue anyway so the menopause has not made a lot of difference."

"It is hard to separate the ME and the menopause which have created emotional distance with partner."

"Sex before the menopause was already prone to being uncomfortable and has become more so since. It hasn't changed

my feelings towards my partner but I do feel avoidant of sex."

"How can I tell my husband that after years of him being patient and understanding that I am uncomfortable or just don't have the energy that now I just don't want to be touched? Some nights I it was ok and I was happy to cuddle but the minute he touched my breasts my skin crawled. I know he felt rejected, he was being rejected. It wasn't constant either, it was only sometimes. I ended up making excuses, I had a headache or I was too tired rather than the real reason. Actually at those times everything about him irritates me and I know it is not his fault. It was easier once I realized that this was happening because as hard as it was I could try and take a step back and look at it objectively. I had to bite my tongue and try and be kind about how I felt rather than rip his head off."

"My libido and energy levels have been up and down. Sometimes I want more intimacy and others I have no interest at all, and then I would do anything to avoid."

"Since I first became ill with ME I have had to try and balance my life to include sex. It frequently left me tired and drained for the next day or so. I know that if I choose to have sex I will have to sacrifice something else because it drains me physically and mentally. It is difficult to explain this to my husband because I sometimes think "If we have sex now I won't be able to do x, y or z later." It's not that I don't want to but I know it is at the expense of something else."

"Sex was very painful at the onset of the menopause due to extreme dryness. I think my partner feels rejected which has caused tension and distance between us."

"If I don't schedule sex for a time during the day I am often too

tired or in too much pain at night. My partner feels I'm rejecting him even though I try to not to. I don't know whether I am more tired because of the menopause or just that I am having a bad week or month, it's hard to tell. I definitely not as interested in having sex as I used to be most of the time but my libido hasn't disappeared completely. I'm more irritable too which doesn't make me feel like sex at all."

Sleep disorders

This can include disturbed sleep, insomnia (not being able to sleep), restless leg syndrome, sleep apnea, snoring and narcolepsy. The average adult needs approximately 7-8 hours undisturbed sleep per night. Not getting this can lead to a weakened immune system.

Symptoms can include wakening several times a night, taking more than half an hour to fall asleep, sleep walking or talking, snoring loudly, choking or gasping, and feelings of paralysis on waking. Night sweats can disrupt sleep patterns. Sleep disorders can lead to depression and anxiety which then complete the cycle by making it difficult to sleep. Lack of sleep can also affect our immune system, can make us irritable (affecting our relationships), lead us to gain weight and making it difficult to concentrate or communicate properly. Sleep apnea rates rise sharply after the menopause and affects around 9% of postmenopausal women. During the time from menopausal to postmenopausal insomnia rates in women rise by around 40% with 41% reporting waking up frequently during the night and approximately 16% of postmenopausal women reporting having trouble falling asleep.

What are the causes?

Declining levels of oestrogen and progesterone affects sleep. When oestrogen levels decline it slows down the intake and production of magnesium (this mineral helps the muscles to relax), it also produces night sweats which can interrupt sleep patterns. Declining oestrogen levels have been linked to sleep apnea. Progesterone has a sleep inducing effect on the body and as its levels decline we may find it more difficult to fall asleep.

Stress and anxiety may make it difficult to fall asleep but waking early in the morning can be caused by depression.

What treatments are there?

Try to have a daily routine and time for getting up and only go to bed when you are sleepy. There is no point lying awake and becoming frustrated. Avoid stimulants such as alcohol, caffeine, spicy food and nicotine. Try to limit your fluid intake during the evenings to avoid waking up needing the toilet in the middle of the night. Try practising relaxation techniques to relax your body and mind. Alternative therapies such as aromatherapy, massage or hypnosis can calm the mind and promote sleep. Exercise and fresh air can also help us sleep better, a short walk before bed might help you drop off more easily. When researching I found that the recommended temperature for bedroom can be anything from 65 -72 degrees Fahrenheit which is 18.3-22.2 Celsius for menopausal women.

There are herbal as well as pharmaceutical options available which can help in the short term but if the problem becomes severe you should consider consulting your doctor. There are a variety of medication that can be prescribed which may help in the short term.

ME sufferers and sleep

I asked the volunteers "Has the menopause affected your sleep patterns?" and the response broke down as follows

57% Yes
43% No, not really
Included in those who answered yes 14% said they were unable to sleep although 7% already suffered with insomnia before the

menopause. Also 38% attributed their difficulties sleeping with night sweats and hot flushes which also left them drained.

Disturbed sleep can feel even more devastating to someone who already feels exhausted and tried. Women who suffer from ME will usually need more sleep and rest than the average person so this can be a real problem. Clearly trying to address the issue of hot flushes and night sweats will help a large proportion of women and this is covered in the chapters Hot Flushes.

It may be necessary to change when you sleep. This is why keeping a record of when you have more energy and plan around that rather than trying to force sleep at night. While it is better to sleep at night and have as "normal" routine as possible it is better to have good quality sleep at any time than none at all.

The MEA survey actually rated relaxation as the best treatment when looking at what was most effective closely followed by sleep hygiene clinics although they did comment on the lack of availability of this.

"When I have night flushes it means I don't sleep"

"I have insomnia with night sweats and one of the main factors of NOT feeling well and having ME symptoms the next day is lack of sleep and in this way the menopause affects me greatly."

"Before I slept too much now, due to anxiety symptoms I have very broken sleep at night."

"I get very little sleep most days then sleep for about a week at once just waking to eat or wash etc"

"I sometimes wake due to the intensity of hot flushes and feelings of vertigo."

Weight

Approximately 90% of menopausal women experience some weight gain during this time. Typically between the ages of 45-55 the average woman's weight gain is 12-15lbs. This is when most women experience the menopause and is usually spread around their middle rather than spread all over. Typically when a woman gains weight during the menopause she gains it around her middle. The hour glass figure is lost and a spare tyre appears. Ideally the ratio of the waist to hips should measure less than 0.8 (waist measurement divided by the hip measurement). Higher than this and it increases your risk of cancer (especially breast cancer because of the extra oestrogen being produced), heart disease, high blood pressure, Type 2 diabetes, stroke and Alzheimer's. According to the Menopause Matters website "Women who gain in excess of 20 pounds after the menopause **increase their breast cancer risk** by nearly 20 percent, but those who lose 20 pounds after menopause reduce their breast cancer risk by as much as 23 percent"

What causes this?

As we get older our metabolic rate slows meaning that we need fewer calories before we gain weight.

Our hormone levels change which can affect the way we store fat. As we enter the menopause the ovaries produce less oestrogen so the body looks for alternative sources. A woman's body will work hard to convert calories into fat as fat cells can produce oestrogen. This causes weight gain because fat cells don't burn calories as quickly as muscle cells do.

A woman's body may feel heavier and she might feel to gain inches because as progesterone levels reduce water weight and bloating increase due to water retention. The hormone levels of Androgen increase during the menopause. This sends a message to send to the mid-section instead of the hips. This area around the middle is effective at using the fat cells to produce oestrogen and is the body's way of trying to balance dropping levels. Testosterone helps create lean muscle mass and as its levels drop fewer calories are turned into muscle mass. As muscle cells burn more calories than fat cells the metabolic rate drops.

There is a lot made about people being insulin resistant and this is the reason high protein diets work. They work on the principle that eating carbohydrates will cause your pancreas to secrete excess insulin, and as insulin is involved in the storage of fat, excess fat will be stored in your fat cells. There are actually only a small percentage of people who are insulin resistant but we will produce excess insulin and therefore excess fat if we over-eat carbohydrates. Exercise can help your body utilized both insulin and glucose and while many people lose weight on high protein diets that is often because you consume less calories as you protein takes longer to digest.

There is a decrease of approximately 5% in a woman's metabolic rate per decade and by the time a woman is in her late 40's she may need 200 fewer calories just to maintain her weight. According to one study the drops in oestrogen and progesterone levels can actually *increase* a woman's appetite, causing her to eat up to 67% more. It is no wonder than many women find it so easy to put weight on and so hard to lose it or that the number of women over weight jumps 12% when comparing those in their 40's to those in their 20's and 30's.

What can I do to prevent this?

Clearly diet plays a large part in winning this battle with the bulge.

Exercise is helpful too. Not only does it mean that you are burning more calories through physical exertion but by building muscle mass you can increase the calorific burn further. Muscle cells burn more calories than fat cells; therefore by building muscle instead of fat you are staying healthier, and making your body more efficient. Studies have shown that while some women did put on weight when taking HRT, the same number lost weight so it clearly depends on the individual.

"I have put on over a stone yet I eat less"

"It made me gain a lot of weight initially and crave sugar and carbs."

"I am finding it more difficult to lose weight but cannot be sure that it is caused by the menopause."

"It hasn't changed my eating habits but I have put on about a stone in the last 13 years or so. If I don't take care my weight would keep on creeping upwards. I guess slowed metabolism means I need less food to remain at my ideal weight (unfortunately). I've tried and am trying (rather half-heartedly) now. But as I'm not overweight my motivation to lose half a stone or so hasn't been strong enough to succeed – so far!"

"I eat more now and have put on weight."

"I put a stone on very quickly when I first became ill and since then I gain weight very easily. I think I found it difficult to adapt from being an active person who could burn off food easily to putting weight on. Since the menopause I have found it harder to lose weight even when I cut back on what I am eating and not being able to exercise makes it doubly hard."

As women with ME we are automatically at a disadvantage when it comes to losing weight because the ability to exercise is limited or non-existent. Gaining weight can often be easier than losing weight although some women can lose weight when they initially become ill. Clearly if you can pre-empt any weight gain by eating a healthy diet then you won't have to face the battle of losing the excess lbs.

It may also be helpful to try and define it there are any reasons for you to overeat. We often use food as a crutch or eat emotionally. The conflicting feelings about being ill and the huge changes it can have on your life may be something that you still haven't dealt with so you are using food to either ignore those issues or to replace what you feel to have lost. The menopause can seem like another major event in your life, marking that you are getting older, that you may not have any more children and that time is running out. Some women feel they are outliving their usefulness as children leave home. It is easy to say be positive, imagine the peace and quiet at home, the relief at knowing you won't be faced with the sleepless nights and nappies that more children would bring but not everybody can feel that way and food is an easy way to make yourself feel better. Certain foods increase your endorphins giving you a short term high which can easily be replaced with another chocolate bar when you start to feel low again. I am not saying that this is the case for everyone but if you are consistently gaining weight and you feel powerless when it comes to food then perhaps there is a reason behind it.

I totally agree with Dr Shepherd's view that people with ME have enough restrictions on their lives without following strict diets but I don't think he is advocating an "eat as much as you can" free-for-all. As we are aware from the endless items in the news obesity levels in society are rising and there is an increase in related health problems. Additional health problems are something nobody wants and which would you prefer? To carry on eating too much of the wrong foods and endure other illnesses as well as your ME or making some changes in your diet and learn to manage the illness you have to the best of your ability?

Please refer to the chapters on diet and exercise for further reading.

Diet

Eating well for the menopause

It is important to maintain a healthy diet whatever your age. For women going through the menopausal weight gain is inevitable if you continue eating the same diet due to the slowing of your metabolism. Also you may be much less active either just through your lifestyle as well as your illness.

A variety of digestive problems seem to be associated with ME/CFS although we don't really know why. There are also a lot of sufferers who seem to suffer from allergies or intolerances, particularly to dairy products and wheat. This may be a coincidence but the effects can range from mild to extremely debilitating. IBS (Irritable Bowel Syndrome) is also something which many sufferers experience.

I have read a great deal about diet during the menopause and diet for ME/CFS sufferers. There seems to be a new diet or super food every other week in the press which will help you through the menopause. It can be very confusing. I have broken it down very basically here for you.

Calcium

It is important to make sure you have enough Calcium in your diet. We need sufficient vitamin D in our diet to help with bone development and calcium absorption. We do not get vitamin D from food but from sunlight so for people suffering from ME who may be housebound it is worth considering taking a supplement. Low-fat dairy products, sardines, fortified orange juice, almonds and even some mineral waters contain calcium. If you diet is low in calcium you can also take supplement although too much calcium can be harmful. A healthy adult needs 800mg but over 50's are recommended of 1200mg total calcium in their diet including supplements. This is important to help protect your bones.

Carbohydrates

Carbohydrates are the main source for our energy supply and someone who is physically very active needs more carbohydrates. Equally someone who is ill or leads a very sedentary lifestyle needs less. There are two types of carbohydrates, refined such as white bread, white pasta, sugar, cakes, sweets, sugar, syrup, white pasta and rice and unrefined such as whole grains, brown rice, whole meal pasta, unrefined oats, unsweetened fruit juices, and potatoes. When food is refined it removes protein, minerals, B vitamins, vegetable oils and fibre. Fibre is important for your digestive system so try to eat less refined bread and pasta and switch to wholegrain varieties. Eat plenty of fruit, vegetables, beans, peas and legumes, nuts and seeds. More fibre in your diet can help lower cholesterol, lower blood pressure and relieve constipation. The complex carbohydrates in whole grains, potatoes (with skins), unrefined oats and brown rice are slower to digest so they have a slower effect on blood glucose compared to refined carbohydrates (which are pure sugar or starch and can lead to low blood sugars in some people).

Protein

Protein contains amino acids which the body uses for the repair and replacement of all body cells. Protein can be found in fish, meat, eggs and dairy products but also in nuts, seeds, vegetables, beans and grains which do not contain the saturated fats of animal based proteins. Protein is essential for making anti-bodies, for the neurotransmitters and the hormones and chemicals produced by the immune system. They are also important for recovery from illness because we need a good intake of amino acids. Some of these can be made in our bodies but the essential amnio acids have to come from our diet and it is essential that the protein supplies all of the 12 essential amino acids.

Proteins from animal sources such as meat, fish, milk products and eggs contain all of these in the right balance while the plant based proteins are not. This can be overcome by combining plant proteins such as lentils and rice or wheat with beans.

The best sources of animal based protein are

- Seafood and fish – this is usually low in fat (oily fish is higher but it is a healthier Omega 3 fatty acids)
- White meat poultry – the white meat is leaner as the dark meat contains more fat. The skin is high in saturated fat.
- Dairy products – this included milk, cheese and yogurt. It is also good for your bones. Skimmed and low fat varieties are still good for bone health but better for controlling weight
- Eggs
- Pork tenderloin – this is a leaner cut of meat
- Lean beef – with the emphasis on lean. A similar size piece of skinned chicken breast has only 1gram less saturated fat than lean beef.

The best sources of plant based protein are

- Beans – kidney beans, pinto beans, soy beans, black beans. Half a cup of beans can contain as much protein as a 90gram piece of grilled steak. They will also keep you full as they are full of fibre.
- Soya – Tofu is also low in fat
- Non dairy milk – such as soy and almond milk

- Vegetables – such as avocado, broccoli, peas, spinach, cooked sweat potatoes and kale
- Nuts and seeds – such as cashew, sesame, walnut, almonds, pistachio, peanuts (including nut butters like peanut butter)
- Grains – Brown rice, wheat germ, bulgar wheat, oat bran, oatmeal, quinoa, arnarantha

Some people who are allergic to cow's milk can tolerate goat's or sheep's milk. Soya is an alternative however intolerance to this can develop easily in people who prone to allergies. There are more and more products on the market now that are lactose free for those who have an intolerance and medication which can help. The best person to ask about this is your doctor as there may be side-effects or they may interact with other medication.

Ensure that you are drinking enough water. Not only does it help eliminate toxins from the body but it also hydrates the skin and the cells.

FATS

Remember that your body does need some fat. We need to ensure we have the right balance of fats, ensuring that we have more essential fats and less saturated fat. Essential fatty acids are found in fish (especially oily fish), nuts and seeds, vegetables and good quality polyunsaturated margarines and vegetable oils. The body does not produce these are they have to come from what we eat. They are vital for all body function as they form the main structure of the walls and membranes of all our body cells. Our nerves have an insulating coat composed of fatty acids (myelin sheath) and 80% of the white matter of our brain is made from essential fatty acids.

The two main groups of fatty acids are saturated and unsaturated fats. Saturated fats are mainly hard or animal based fats and are found in meat, cheese, butter, lard, hard margarines and overheated oils while unsaturated fats are usually soft or liquid at room temperature. Do be aware that vegetable oils take on hydrogen atoms when heated (such as being used for deep frying) and become saturated. Vegetable oils and hardened margarines which are processed contain saturated fatty acids which actually block the way the body utilizes good essential fats so they can actually be worse for you than butter and cream.

One role of Essential Fatty Acids is the production of PROSTAGLANDINS. These are short-lived in the diet and regulate the biochemistry and enzyme activities in all our cells. It is made from an essential fat found in vegetable oils called linoleic acid.

PGE1 is an important prostaglandin because it improves the blood circulation, lowers blood pressure, inhibits inflammation, restore normal shape and movement of the red blood cells, effects the nerve conduction and transmission at the nerve endings and activate T lymphocytes in the immune system. If you are deficient in vitamin B6, zinc, magnesium and biotin it can block the production of PGE1, as can diabetes, alcohol, chemicals and viral infections. Taking Gamma Linolenic Acid directly into the diet can bypass any blockage and can be found in Evening Primrose Oil, Starflower Oil or Blackcurrant Seed Oil.

PGE2 is another prostaglandin which promotes clotting in the blood, narrowing of the blood vessels, swelling and inflammation. This also comes from linoleic acid, via arachidonic acid, which also occurs in meat. A diet with less meat but more fish and vegetables will produce more PGE1 which is anti-inflammatory whereas a diet high in meat will produce more PGE2 which is pro-inflammatory.

PGE3 is important for preventing thrombosis and are made from alpha-linolenic acids, found in beans, wheat and spinach, and eicosapentanoeic acid (EPA) which is found in fish oils.

Dr Anne Macintyre advises people with ME/CFS (particularly if they have allergies) take both GLA, as EPO or blackcurrant seed oil, and EPA as fish oil.

Therefore we must learn to have a good balance of fats if we are to manage both our ME/CFS and the menopause. We are bombarded by adverts that tell us about low fat and fat free products. As you will see from above, our bodies need fat in our diet but we need the right fats and the right balance of fats.

Debra Waterhouses, author of "Menopause without Weight Gain", advises that a diet of fat free foods does not enable your menopausal body to function well.

Soy is beneficial for women going through the menopause because they contain plant oestrogens which help relieve some menopausal symptoms.

Bloating

This can be another symptom of the menopause and is usually caused by water retention, intestinal gas or a mixture of the two. It can be due to fluctuating hormones and sometimes weight gain. It can lead to an uncomfortable tightness or fullness in the stomach. Swallowing too much air, carbonated drinks, IBS and a change in diet can create intestinal gas (so can lactose intolerance). One of the side effects of HRT can be bloating.

Foods, such as, fruit juices and herbal teas, yogurt and hard cheese, eggs, rice, peanut butter, bananas and grapes have been shown to reduce bloating.

Diet, ME and the menopause

Some of the women who wrote to me have managed to improve both their weight issues and some of their ME symptoms by adjusting their diets, in particular identifying some allergies that have been aggravating their symptoms. Many have eliminated dairy, wheat and sugar from their diets and have found that helps. The MEA survey shows that others have found allergy treatments, vitamins/supplements and EPA Omega 3 oil have helped with their ME symptoms.

For a healthy menopause without weight gain I do believe that it is about finding a good balance of quality and quantity. We need to be careful not only about what we are eating but the amounts. We need to be supplying out bodies with variation of good quality food without overeating. Any diet will only work as long as you stick to it, whether you are ill or not. I agree with Dr Charles Shepherd's view that ME puts enough restrictions on its sufferers without adding a whole range of foods to it.

For someone who loves my food this echoes my feelings but, and it is a big but, if I eat the same amount as when I was active I know I will put weight on. Food for me is a social occasion as well as just enjoyable for the pure taste. It is a treat, a celebration, something to make me feel better. I have had to be very honest about the fact that for years I over ate. I am still prone to it, I enjoy the way food makes me feel. What I don't enjoy are all the side effects from carrying extra weight. The back ache, the way I look (and then feel about myself), the difficulty performing simple tasks which are easier if I am a smaller size. A times food has been compensation too, I might not be able to do the things I want but I can enjoy this chocolate bar, or maybe even two! Food fills an emotional need in me especially when I am having a relapse. My brain tells me "You need energy. Food gives you energy. So eat!"

I recommend reading 'Menopause without Weight Gain' by Debra Waterhouse who goes to great pains to remind us that women going through the menopause are unlikely to achieve the same weight/body shape that they had in their 20's. It is unrealistic for those who are well so I think it is nearly impossible for those of us who are ill and have a limit on their activity levels. We cannot stop the aging process but we can learn to adapt both our lifestyles and our mental approach to it. We can choose to stay as we are or to change if we think it is worth it. Her advice on portion size may come as a surprise to many of you.

If weight gain is an issue for you, try reducing the quantities that you eat. If you image that your stomach is only the size of your clenched fist, and then compare it next to your dinner plate I guarantee you are eating more than will fill your stomach. Eat low calorie foods which fill you up and cut down on, if you can't eliminate, the empty calories. Try using a smaller plate and don't just build it into a skyscraper of food on a plate.

I often see people who are desperate to lose weight and want me to perform a hypno-gastric band hypnotherapy session. They are willing to make changes in their lives to achieve a healthy life and weight. The successful ones look forward to embracing a new life with a new body shape and not because of a new body shape. The problem is that I also see people who want to lose weight but do nothing different to achieve this. I had one client whose requirements were that she wanted to lose 2 stone in 2 months so she could be slim for her birthday. After asking about her diet and life style I asked if she thought that perhaps she could incorporate some more exercise into her day (she didn't like walking or exercise), if she could think of any way to reduce the quantities she was eating (i.e. only have one biscuit instead of 6 with her tea) which she didn't want to do. In truth she wanted to change nothing in her life but she wanted to be thin and she wanted a way where I "fixed it for her". Unfortunately no-one can wave a magic wand and "fix" things for you. You have to want to change. You have to want to lose weight or maintain a healthy weight, and you have to want it more than an extra piece of cake. People who undergo major weight loss surgery *have* to change their lifestyle afterwards. If they continue to overeat their stomach will stretch again and they will gain weight and may cause themselves more damage because of it.

I am not a diet expert. I am not stick thin and, yes, I could do with losing some more weight. I know how difficult losing and managing your weight can be. I also know how difficult I find it to maintain a stable weight with this illness. When I am feeling ill or am having a bad day I eat more than I should do. These are also the days when I do less so I am burning fewer calories. So not only am I prone to put weight on when I am having a relapse, I am prone to putting it on quickly. If you then consider that as my metabolic rate is dropping due to age and the menopause I will need even less calories my future weight looked guaranteed to increase if I am not careful. I am not saying that everyone with ME is the same as me in this respect. Some people don't feel like eating when they are ill and actually lose weight.

It is easy to let your weight spiral out of control and quick weight loss plans with restrictive diets are not the answer. Not only will you put the weight back on when you go back to normal but they are not recommended for people suffering from ME. They can make you feel drained and may even prompt a relapse especially if you suddenly try to start exercising and push yourself too far. Therefore a balance diet as a way of life is a better approach especially if you can reduce your portion size. Almost all diets that you read about or try will work if you can stick at them and not return to your old eating habits. It may be slower to simply make healthier choices and reduce the amount you eat but it is a healthier approach. It is less likely to aggravate your illness too.

I know that every diet tells you that this one is a new way of life, a new easy way of life. I would love to be able to tell you that changing your diet for a few weeks is the answer to your weight problems but it isn't. Make small changes by choosing healthier options and smaller portions. It may be worth weighing some food so you can see how much a healthy size portion of your chosen food is. I was amazed at how small an amount we actually need. Keeping a food diary will show you just how much you are really eating. We usually under-estimate how much we really eat.

Having a good diet filled with good healthy food can only be good for you. A varied diet will give you the vitamins and minerals you need to stay healthy as well control your weight.

Exercise

Exercise is important to keep us healthy. Combined with a healthy diet it you can prevent main health risks associated with the menopause, heart disease and osteoporosis. It can also help lower blood pressure, prevent Type 2 diabetes, aid the digestive system which can alleviate constipation and boost your immune function.

Exercise can help strengthen your heart and lungs. It also helps to lower cholesterol levels, increase good cholesterol HDL and lower bad cholesterol LDL. Exercise can help control chronic inflammation, heart disease and degenerative conditions such as arthritis. Inflammation is connected to illnesses.

Exercise when combined with a healthy diet can halve the risk of developing Type 2 diabetes.

It can boost your immune function and keeping active can help ward off colds. One study showed that women who walked for 30 minutes a day had half the number of colds when compared to those who were physically inactive. Walking the same amount has been shown to half the risk of developing breast cancer and reduces the risk of bowl cancer by up to a quarter independent of obesity, smoking and diet. Exercise provides beneficial effects.

The lymphatic system filters out waste and accumulated bacteria. This relies on movement rather than a pump like a heart to move the lymph, a water yellowish fluid, around the body. The lymphatic system is important in the detoxification and immune function of the body.

All the research shows that it is the total amount of exercise that is important rather than the type or intensity. Clearly for people suffering from any illness where fatigue is predominant feature this is difficult. Finding a balance of what you are capable of will depend very much on what stage you at with you illness. If you are having a period of acute ME or a relapse then exercise may not be possible or advisable so please consult your doctor before beginning any form of exercise.

Exercises can be done in small sections. Half an hours' walking could be broken down into three 10 minute walks. If you start to feel tired, STOP. There is no benefit to managing a half an hour walk to then be ill for a week. Never push yourself to exhaustion. Know your limits and be prepared to readjust the amount and type of exercise according to how you are each day. Little and often can still be beneficial. Of course even this may not be achievable if the simple act of getting dressed leaves you completely drained but during your better spells you will still benefit from doing something, no matter how small.

There is a danger when you feel well enough to try something energetic, only to be forced to stop after a short time and possibly even cause another relapse. This is something that is echoed again and again by experts so it is an important piece of advice. Do not push yourself too far or too hard. The 'no pain, no gain' mind set does not help sufferers of ME, it hinders them.

Here are some precautions that you can take to help avoid a relapse.

- Walking circular routes then you will be heading back home rather than get stranded
- Walk routes that have somewhere to sit and rest if you need to
- Carry a mobile phone with you or take a companion who can fetch the car if needed

- When swimming try to find a pool with warmer water (some pools hold special sessions for people with illness where the temperature is warmer)
- Try exercises such as yoga or Thai chi which involve gentle stretching
- Set your own pace and stop before you get tired
- Remember your energy levels may vary greatly. Just because you could do something yesterday it doesn't mean you'll be able to do it today or tomorrow
- Try stretching exercises that you can do while lying in bed.
- Only attempt to increase the intensity, duration and frequency of exercise very slowly. If necessary only increase it by a minute a week and be prepared to cut back if you experience any symptoms
- Rest after exercise, even if only briefly, to let your body recover

Stretching exercises seem to be well tolerated by people with ME/CFS especially as these can be done in bed. Yoga incorporates this and seems to be popular choice with sufferers. Swimming is also good as the water offers some support, putting less strain on the joints and muscles although cold water can aggravate muscle pain. The water also offers resistance and you can exercise both your upper and lower body at the same time. Walking is a cheap form of exercise with the benefits of getting you out in the fresh air. Lack of exercise can lead to muscle wastage so even doing small exercises while sitting down can help prevent this.

Learn from any relapses. Try to keep a diary to find out what works for you and what doesn't. If walking for 20 minutes causes a relapse do not assume you can't walk. Reduce it to 5 minutes and if you are ok with that and do it every other day. If that causes problems cut back further. If you can do 5 minutes try increasing it to 10mins one day and then if you have no adverse effects add an extra 5 minutes on an in-between day. Only increase the intensity, duration and frequency SLOWLY. If necessary increase it one minute at a time and ALWAY STOP BEFORE YOU GET TIRED.

Remember to vary your activity levels according to your energy levels. Also varying the type of exercise is not only good for your body but will stop it feeling like a chore. If you don't feel up to exercising one day, then don't.

Yoga

Yoga has been rated quite highly by volunteers in the MEA survey although it clearly isn't for everyone. There seem to be more and more clinics and workshops aimed at people with ME which use a variety of approaches and yoga is often listed among them. It is a gentle form of exercise which also promotes relaxation and calm. It is often used with mediation which scored 2nd to pacing in the best management strategy in their study. Exercising the muscles as well as promoting a healthy mental state can help with both the menopause and ME symptoms. It might also be fun and help you to meet new people.

Graded Exercise Therapy (GET)

This is something which was widely used to help ME/CFS sufferers by the NHS. This is where exercise levels increased gradually but unfortunately this has actually been shown to make some people worse instead of better. In the 2010 MEA it rated bottom in the treatments that sufferers felt had helped with over half reporting that it had made them worse. This is why it is so important to be extremely careful when approaching any form of exercise and, in my opinion, you have to learn to listen to your body and not overdo any exercise which may cause a relapse.

Exercise – For and against

Walking

You can choose your own route	You can overtire yourself and get too far from home
You are out in the fresh air	Temperature – can be too hot or cold
It is cheap. No expense except shoes	You may need someone to be with you
You can meet other people (social interaction is good)	You may get waylaid by well meaning people

Swimming

Water supports the body (putting less strain on the muscles and joints)	Getting to the pool can be tiring
Resistance of water makes movements effective	Cold water can aggravate muscle pain
You can meet people and socialize	Cost
You can set your own pace	You may need help getting changed

Yoga

It is a gentle form of exercise	Must be careful not to overstretch
Helps with posture and balance	May have to avoid some positions (especially upside down ones)

Can be done at home	May need to attend classes to learn correct positions
Socializing (if attending classes)	Cost

Thai Chi

A gentle form of exercise	Must not overstretch
Helps both the body and the mind	May need help learning movements
Can be done at home	Cost of classes
Can socialize if attending classes	Attending classes can be tiring

Computer Programs (E.g. Wii-fit, Xbox 360, PS)

You can pick and choose which exercises to do	You have to motivate yourself
You can specify the length of the session	Sound effects can be aggravating if you are sensitive to noises
Can be played with family/friends	Other family members might take it over
Can choose time (day or night)	You don't meet new people

HRT – Hormone Replacement Therapy

What is HRT?

A woman's ovaries stop producing the hormones oestrogen and progesterone around the time of the menopause. HRT is a treatment which replaces these hormones and is proven to help treat hot flushes and vaginal discomfort.

The loss of oestrogen, in both the long and short term, is the causes of menopausal symptoms. The synthetic form of progestogen in HRT helps protect the lining of the womb and protect changes which may develop in to cancer.

Bio-identical hormones are more effectively used by the body with fewer side-effects than synthetic hormones. Bio-identical (or natural) hormones come from plant sources such as soy and wild yams. They will not produce the same side-effects or increase the risk of cancer caused by synthetic hormones as they contain a molecular structure that is identical (or bio-identical) to that of the hormones produced by the human body. They are useful to the female body by relieving the symptoms of the menopause.

Synthetic hormones are not natural but are manufactured in laboratories. They can produce side-effects such as water retention, dizziness and nausea. They also carry the potential risks of cancer (breast and uterine).

The history of HRT

HRT (Hormone Replacement Therapy) is prescribed to relief menopausal symptoms. It has been available from the 1940s but became more commonly used in the 1960s. Concerns were raised regarding the safety of HRT after the publication of two studies in

2002 and 2003. There were two main areas of concern, the first being that if used for an extended period of time HRT may increase the risk of breast cancer and secondly that the risk of heart disease may increase with the use of HRT.

1940s HRT became available

1960s HRT became more commonly used

1993 WHI (Women's Health Initiative) looked at the health effect of HRT on women. A clinical trial in the US compared women taking combined HRT or oestrogen only HRT to women taking a placebo.

1996 Million Women Study started collecting questionnaire in the UK on HRT use and the effects that it had on certain issues of women's health.

2002 The study by the WH into combined (oestrogen and progesterone) HRT was stopped early after findings raised concerns due to a small increased risk of heart disease, breast cancer, blood clots and stroke. The results were published in 2003.

2003 Many women stop taking HRT and doctors advise patients to come off HRT as they are confused about the safety issue which is hyped up by the media.

2004 The oestrogen only part of the WHI study finds trends for beneficial effects on heart disease and breast cancer but still a small increase in the risk of stroke.

2003-2007 HRT users more than halves from 2 million to less than a million in the UK.

2004-2007 WHI publishes more analysis of their trial which shows that some safety issues were over-estimated in their 2002 findings. It shows additional benefits for those starting HRT between the age of 50-59 or those who are less than 10 years past the menopause. There was a trend to a lower risk from both heart disease and death from any cause with no clear increase risk of stroke in this group. For those starting HRT after 60 years of age it did show a general increased risk.

WISDOM (Women's International Study of long Duration Oestrogen after the Menopause) had many of the same findings concerning the increased risk of heart disease particularly in older women who began or restarted hormone therapy after the menopause.

Dr Steven Goldstein of North American Menopause Society sad "What we discovered is that if a women between the ages of 50 and 55 when she starts taking hormones, or if she begins HRT less than 10 years after she started the menopause, she has less heart disease and death from any cause, compared to the placebo group."

JAMA (Journal of American Medical Association) published the results of research in 2007. Their report did say that the risk of stroke in some users increased by up to 32% regardless of age or years since the menopause.

The New England Journal of Medicine published similar research, looking at younger women who had a hysterectomy and took oestrogen alone, in June 2008 reinforcing this and suggesting that HRT may have a positive effect on the heart.

The JAMA report also showed that the women (who had hysterectomies and oestrogen only therapy for an average of 7 years) had no increase in the rates of breast cancer; in fact risks of one type of breast cancer were reduced in these women.

Some doctors seem to feel that a drop in breast cancers have been, in part, due to a drop in hormone use.

Main Types of HRT

Cyclical or Sequential

This is recommended for women who are still having periods and menopausal symptoms but approaching the menopause or women who have had a natural menopause within the last year. It mimics the menstrual pattern. Oestrogen is taken every day and progestogen is taken in addition for 10-14 days. At the end of the progestogen course as the body withdraws from the hormone a bleed will usually occur. The progestogen protects the lining of the womb from harmful pre-cancerous changes and regulates the bleeding.

Oestrogen-only HRT

This type of HRT is prescribed to women who have had with their womb or womb and ovaries removed by a hysterectomy as progestogen in no longer needed to protect the womb lining.

Continuous Combined HRT or Period-Free HRT

Although spotting or breakthrough bleeding may occur during the first few months this form of HRT is period free. It is recommended for postmenopausal women (those women who have not had a period for at least one year) and is a combination of oestrogen and progestogen which is taken every day. Women usually start on cyclical HRT and change to this method later.

Local HRT

This raises hormones in the required area but not the whole body. It is used to treat problems such a vaginal dryness. It can be taken as tablets, creams, peccaries and rings which when inserted into the vagina provide oestrogen that helps reduce vaginal dryness.

Tibolone

This is taken in continuous tablet form and is a synthetic form of period free HRT which provides the similar benefits to oestrogen.

Long Cycle HRT

This type of HRT only causes withdrawal bleeding every 3 months instead of every month and is best suited if a woman sufferers side effects when taking progestogen. There are some questions as to its safety concerning the lining of the womb if taken long term.

HRT is not generally recommended for women who have had breast or endometrial cancer, a stroke or deep-vein blood clot or have severe liver disease.

Side-effects of HRT

The common side effects of HRT are breast tenderness, irregular bleeding and feeling bloated but these are usually mild and resolve themselves in a few months. Side effects can sometimes be reduced by using lower doses of hormones. It is important to discuss any concerns with your doctor.

Benefits of HRT

HRT reduces menopausal symptoms by replacing oestrogen as the levels drop in a woman's body due to the menopause. Within a short time of starting HRT the symptoms of hot flushes and nights sweats usually improve dramatically. This in turn should help reduce insomnia, tiredness and irritability. Many women also find that HRT is beneficial psychologically as it can help with problems such as loss of interest in sex, difficulty in remembering things, concentration, anxiety and depression, over-sensitivity, tearfulness and feelings of irritability and disturbed sleep.

Overview

HRT was at one time hailed as a fountain of youth, a wonder drug that could eliminate the symptoms of the menopause and the aging process. It was quite common for women to continue taking HRT for decades, almost indefinitely. We now know that this isn't a safe course of action. Our age and the length of time taking HRT can have serious implications. It does delay the process of the menopause by replacing the hormones that our bodies are no longer producing. It is useful for reducing symptoms but it is not ideal for everyone. Whether it is right for you will depend on your medical history and your age. It is not something which you can take forever.

I was advised to take HRT initially as I was only in my early 40s when my blood tests confirmed that I was entering an early menopause. I could see the sense in protecting my bones (especially as I wasn't especially active due to my ME) plus my doctor advised me that it would help restore my libido which was galloping away into the distance at an alarming rate of knots. The thought of something which would stop the mood swings that had me snapping everyone's head off with the added benefit of slowly the aging process and the ever increasing wrinkles appealed to me even though I had always presumed I would try and go through this stage of my life naturally when the time came to it. The problem was that I wasn't expecting it to get there quite this quickly. At that time there were celebrities all saying that they had more energy than ever, looking beautiful and radiant. I wanted to feel better. I wanted to be vibrant, sexy and energetic instead of lethargic, moody and old with the sex drive of a comatose sloth.

Unfortunately for me within a month I discovered a lump in my breast. After a trip to the hospital they discovered I had not one but five cysts in one breast and was advised against restarting the treatment. The worrying fact to me was that I could only feel one of the five cysts (being small busted anyway I didn't think there was room for five let alone not being able to detect them!) so I followed their advice. As they pointed out, I was still going to have to go through the menopause so it was either now or when I came off the HRT. The HRT may have eased the symptoms but it was just putting the menopause off for a while. The only sensible option was to deal with the menopause without HRT. I have personally found natural alternatives have had a positive effect so far with all of my symptoms but it has been a case of trial and error.

There are many good reasons for deciding to take HRT and some women feel much better for it but it is best to be advised by your doctor and to read as much as possible about it to ensure that you feel that this is the right course of action for you. It does appear from the responses that I have had that some women have to try several different types before they find one that suits them. Personally I think that I would find this tiring but if your symptoms are extreme perhaps it is a better option.

I am not advising women for or against taking HRT. As with

everything with this illness I believe that it can be individual to each of us. You have to find what works best for you.

Alternative therapies

Healing Crisis

What is a healing crisis? You will often hear this mentioned as a result of alternative therapy treatments. This can range from a mild sniffle to headaches. It also is usually a feeling of tiredness and the patient may feel emotional afterward. This is normal and is usually when they are thought to be 'letting go' and releasing either toxins from the body or and build up of emotions in a healthy way. This rarely lasts more than 24 hours and your energy levels and feelings of wellbeing should then return. It is also advisable to stay hydrated by drinking plenty of water, to avoid exercise and heavy fatty or sugary foods (and alcohol) during the first 24 hours. If you have any concerns about how you will feel after a treatment make sure you ask the practitioner to explain what you should expect before they begin and plan for an easy 24 hours after treatments.

Acupuncture and acupressure

What is it?

Acupuncture involves inserting small fine needles into certain points on the body. Based on ancient Chinese medicine it works on the principle that energy channels around the body (meridians) can become blocked and pain can be removed by clearing them. Acupressure involved the manipulation of these points using pressure rather than inserting needles.

Common uses

It is used for a wide variety of issues. Headache, migraine, back and neck pain, joint, dental and post operative pain, allergies, fatigue, depression and anxiety, digestive problems such as IBS, and insomnia to mention a few.

Side-effects

This treatment is not suitable for people with blood disorders or who are on certain medications that thin the blood. Please check with your doctor before considering this treatment. A small percentage of patients may experience bruising or bleeding, drowsiness or a worsening of pre-existing conditions. These are usually mild and short lived. Acupuncture is safe when conducted by a properly trained practitioner.

Cost and frequency

Initial sessions usually range from £35-60 with subsequent sessions being £25-50. You will usually require between 6 and 12 sessions which will last between 20 and 40 minutes. Prices and session lengths can vary from therapist to therapist. Its use in the NHS is limited so you will generally have to pay for this treatment.

Benefits for ME and the menopause

Some sufferers find that this therapy can help them manage both the pain that they have due to ME and some symptoms caused by the menopause. Several women have commented specifically that it has helped balance out hot flushes, headaches and other associated symptoms of both the menopause and their ME.

Aromatherapy

What is it?

This therapy uses essential oils which are distilled. They are very concentrated and need to be diluted. They can be inhaled or absorbed through the skin when used either for massage or in the bath. Smells can be mood enhancing and they may be useful for relieving pain and massage is relaxing and beneficial in reducing stress related illnesses. Aromatherapy promotes physical and mental well-being. Some oils have anti-viral properties, while some are general healers. Others affect blood pressure. They are not generally recommended for oral consumption. Massage also speed up the circulation and improve the nourishment of the skin tissues.

Common uses

Oils can be blended and each one has different properties and can help different symptoms. There are certain oils which should be avoided if you have high blood pressure or are pregnant. Not only do they smell nice but they can be used to help a wide (almost endless) range of problems. Essential oils should be diluted as they come in a concentrated form. A few drops in a warm bath or into water either to inhale or heat on an oil burner is all you need. For massage it should be mixed with a base or carrier oil (such as sweet almond, grape, or soya oil) at a ratio of about 20 drops to 100ml of base oil.

Side-effects

Overuse of essential oil can cause headaches and can make you feel unwell. Certain oils should be avoided if you are pregnant as it can cause bleeding or suffer from high blood pressure. You should also avoid certain oils if you have sensitive skin. It is essential to use an experienced aroma-therapist and also ensure that they are aware of any medical problems you have. If you are using them at home please research thoroughly to confirm that it is suitable for you. Also try a test patch rather than use it all over your body to ensure you do not have any adverse effects.

Remember that you can 'overdose' on these if you have a few drops in the bath while using them in a burner followed by an aromatherapy massage and a few drops on your pillow. Choose one method at a time unless you want a headache!

Cost and frequency

Essential oils can start at a few pounds but some can be expensive. If you are having an aromatherapy massage it will depend if you are having a full body, just back and shoulders or sports massage. The time can vary from 30 to 90 minutes and therefore the so can the cost.

Benefits for ME and menopause

It is best to buy oils that have been premixed unless you know what you are doing as over use of an oil can make you feel unwell. Also certain oils blend better together than others. They are easy to use in a burner or in the bath and can help ease your symptoms. A drop or two of lavender on your pillow might help you sleep better but more could have the opposite effect of keeping you awake. An essential oil, if mixed with a carrier oil, and massaged into the skin will not only sooth sore muscles but can improve both your skin and promote the body to release any toxins.

Some oils and their uses

Avocado or wheat germ oil can help dry skin
Juniper, lavender, rosemary oils can help with muscle and joint pain
Lavender, peppermint oils can help with headaches
Basil oil can help with fatigue
Neroli and lavender oil can help with insomnia

Clary sage and rose can help raise a depressed mood

_Bergamot oil is calming and uplifting

Camomile oil can help reduce tension and sleep

Cedar wood oil is soothing

Geranium oil is calm and cooling and is useful for tension

Lavender oil can help with headaches and stimulate the mind

Peppermint oil can relieve decongestion and headaches

Rosemary oil has stimulating effect but should be avoided during pregnancy

Ylang ylang oil has a sedating effect.

Ayurveda

This alternative therapy takes a holistic approach to health and includes a variety of treatments. These include the use of herbs, massage and detoxification. Practitioners are most likely to be found in Asian communities as it is based on an ancient Indian holistic approach, looking at the body as a whole.

CBT (Cognitive Behavioural therapy) and Psychotherapy

What is it?

CBT (Cognitive Behavioural Therapy) and Psychotherapy are talking therapies which help you change the way you think and deal with problems. It aims to change behaviours that are not helpful and sometimes harmful to you as certain behaviours affect certain health problems.

Common uses

It is usually used to treat anxiety and depression but can also be helpful for people dealing with eating disorders, stress, sleep problems, OCD, phobias, post traumatic stress, bipolar and schizophrenia disorders, anger issues, sexual/relationship issues and pain.

Side-effects

A disadvantage rather than a side effect is that this type of treatment does not suit everyone and you have to commit to process. It is not always suitable for people with learning difficulties and more complex mental health issues so it is wise to be guided by your doctor when considering this treatment.

Cost and frequency

This is usually a short term treatment, lasting from approximately 6 weeks to 6 months. It generally consists of one to one sessions once a week, depending on your condition, with each session lasting approximately for 1 hour. This treatment is available on the NHS is referred by your doctor. If you wish to see a CBT privately you can obtain details of accredited practitioners from the British Association for Behavioural and Cognitive Psychotherapies. Session usually cost between £40 and £100.

Benefits for ME and menopause

This type of treatment is not a cure but aims to help you deal with day to day functioning and find ways of coping which in turn can help improve symptoms. This will normally included managing your energy, pain and activity levels, setting goals, establishing routines (especially sleep related) and to support you psychologically. It can help you deal with the evitable changes that illness has on your life.

EFT (Emotional Freedom therapy)

What is it?

This therapy is based on the same energy meridians that are used in acupuncture but without using needles. EFT uses a combination of talking (voicing positive affirmations) and tapping on those various acupuncture points with your finger tips. This can help remove blockages caused by negative emotions, old behavioural patterns/traumas or events and bring the body and mind back into balance which then aids the natural healing process.

Common Uses

It is used for a wide range of issues such as depression, anxiety, stress/panic attacks, self esteem issues, relationship issues, IBS, insomnia, eating/weight related issues, phobias, anger and physical/pain complaints.

Side effects

This therapy does not ask you to relive any past experiences but it is important to ensure you are tapping in the correct places and that the affirmations you make are phrased correctly for it to be effective.

Cost and frequency

Costs vary from practitioner to practitioner and this is not available on the NHS. An initial appointment (where important information is gathered) will usually last approximately 90 minutes followed by appointments of 60 -75 minutes. You may need several sessions as each issue if different but you should be advised by the practitioner as to how many you will need

Benefits for ME and the menopause

This therapy can be used to help with a number of symptoms for both ME and the menopause. By helping to resolve old issues and negative thought patterns and some studies have shown that it has helped with CFS and fibromyalgia sufferers.

Homeopathy

What is it?

It is based on the theory that a substance that can produce symptoms in a healthy person can cure similar symptoms in someone who is sick. This therapy involves using very small doses of medicine, matching its characteristic to the symptoms, to relieve and eliminate the symptoms and problem or particular disorder by stimulating the healing process. It is always a good idea to receive advice from someone trained in this area. This approach has been shown to have some beneficial effect on the symptoms of the menopause. They are derived from herb, mineral, plant, and animal products.

Common uses

It lists a wide range of ailments that it can help, among which menopause is listed. It can be used treat complaints from acne, bites and bruising through to rheumatism, migraines and warts.

Side-effects

They don't usually cause any side-effects as they are heavily diluted but occasionally they can make patients feel worse when they start taking them.

Cost and frequency

This can vary but will usually involve an initial consultation followed by the cost of treatments.

Benefits for ME and menopause

Menopause is one of the conditions listed that can be helped with homeopathy. It can also help with sleeplessness and anxiety. It is advisable to obtain advice from a trainer practitioner who will determine the best course of treatment based on your individual symptoms.

Hydrotherapy

What is it?

Most of these treatments alternate hot and cold water treatments. Hot water increases the blood flow to the skin by dilating the blood vessels. This can last between 5 and 15 minutes depending on the illness and patients condition. Next cold water is used either by showering, douching or sluicing causing the blood vessels to constrict, reducing blood flow which sends the blood back to the heart and purifying the organs such as the liver.

Common uses

It is claimed to eliminate toxins and increasing blood flow through the skin. It forces blood and nourishment to the internal organs before flushing it out again.

Side-effects

This type of treatment should be avoided if you have any form of heart condition as it can put the heart under extreme strain.

Cost and frequency

This is sometimes available on the NHS and if your doctor decides that this may be beneficial is usually 5 or 6 session, each lasting approximately 30 minutes.

Benefits for ME and menopause

This may be unsuitable for ME sufferers who are sensitive to chemicals. Also the heat of the water and exercise may leave you feeling very tired. The heat may also aggravate hot flushes having said that some people find that they are able to move more freely because of the support of the water and the heat is soothing and relaxing for their muscles. However there is a danger that you may overdo any exercise because it feels easier in the water.

Hypnotherapy

What is it?

Hypnosis is a natural state which we all enter several times a day. Hypnotherapy involves placing the client into a state of deep relaxation where the subconscious mind is more open to positive suggestions. The hypnotherapist will make positive suggestions while you are in a hypnotic state so that you can address a wide range of problems or areas that you wish to change in your life. You cannot be forced to do anything against you will and a willingness to make these changes is necessary. It can help you become more accepting of your limitations while encouraging a positive outlook. Many people find that because they enter a deeply relaxed state that they feel better afterwards.

Common uses

Hypnotherapy can be beneficial for dealing with a wide range of issues. These include anxiety and stress, insomnia, overcoming fears and phobias, grief, reducing and managing pain, confidence, weight issues, stopping smoking, motivation, IBS and many more. A good hypnotherapist will always spend time asking you about you background and medical history before any session begins. Hypnotherapy is recommended by NICE for the treatment of IBS. It can also be used to take you back to find an incident that initially caused your problem/issue (even if you are not consciously aware of what it actually was) so that you can identify triggers and make appropriate changes.

Side-effects

When performed by a properly trained therapist there are no side effects and you should simply be left feeling relaxed and refreshed. It is essential that any suggestions made are positive.

Cost and frequency

This is not currently available on the NHS and costs can vary from therapist to therapist. The number of sessions will vary depending on the issues and usually costs between £35-75. Each session will last between 40-60 minutes.

Benefits for ME and menopause sufferers

Hypnotherapy can help deal with issues such as insomnia, IBS, anxiety/depression and regaining self-confidence which can often be lost due to long-term illness. By relaxing the mind and body while making positive suggestions stress and pain can be reduced. Learning to accept the changes you are experiencing, dealing with the loss of your old way of life, staying positive and being focused on positive aspects of your life can improve the overall health/well-being of the client leaving them feeling relaxed and more energized.

A study by the University of Texas and Baynor University has shown that hypnotherapy can reduce menopausal symptoms by up to 75%. It showed a decrease in the frequency of hot flushes of 80%.

Massage

What is it?

Massage is where muscles are rubbed with a variety of different movements such as pummelling, kneading, wringing, knuckling and stroking. It can be effective at freeing the actions of the joints and muscles, stimulating the blood supply and awakening the nerves. The skin contains hundreds of nerves per square centimetre and is sensitive to pain, heat, cold, pressure and touch. When the skin is rubbed with fine oil it can be kept elastic and supple.

Common uses

Not only is massage intensely pleasurable but it can stimulate a sluggish blood supply by forcing the blood vessels to constrict. It can also release stress and tension in the muscles and joints. It also stimulates the lymphatic system encouraging the body to carry waste products from the body and therefore protecting it against infections. It can also help to improve muscle tone.

Side-effects

Basic massage can be carried out at home but for a more intense massage it is best to consult a qualified practitioner or therapist. If oils are used, especially essential oils, care must be taken to consider any existing medical conditions. Also if the muscles are sore or tender and around areas such as various veins massage should either be very gentle or avoided completely.

Cost and frequency

First a full medical history should be taken and your condition assessed. A full body massage will usually last approximately 90 minutes. Prices can vary but usually start around £45 upwards per session. Frequency will depend on you but usually the first few sessions would be once a week. This is not available on the NHS. A back and neck only massage will be quicker and cheaper than a full body.

Benefits for ME and menopause sufferers

Massage can benefit people with ME by releasing stress and tension from the body and relaxing the mind. It can also ease aching muscles and joints as well as stimulating the blood flow and lymphatic system which will encourage the body to release toxins stored in the body. It can help with menopause symptoms in the same way. It can help with muscle tone and the improvement of the skin but care needs to taken if the muscles are sore and tender and at such a time the use of gentle techniques are best.

Reflexology

What is it?

Reflexologists' believe that areas on the foot relate to specific areas in the body and that massaging and manipulating these areas can improve your health. When the corresponding area or zone is massaged it is said to clear any blockages letting the body's energy flow and work as it should. Its origins can be traced back as far as ancient Egypt. India, China and Japan all have their own methods of foot massage.

Common uses

It is commonly used for any condition that needs to be regulated (such as menstrual irregularities), aches and pains, fatigue and stress.

Side-effects

This treatment should not be used on women during the first 3 months of pregnancy. It should not be used to treat diabetes, foot ulcers, gout and other circulatory problems with the feet, thyroid problems and epilepsy. It can also interfere with some medication so please check with your doctor first.

There are very few side-effects with this treatment and if they do occur only usually last for 24 hours. As with many alternative therapies you may have what is referred to as a healing crisis. This may present as cold like symptoms or fatigue, with or without a headache. It is best to stay well hydrated as the elimination of toxins from the body and this can very occasionally result in excess sweating, skin rashes, nausea and thirst. Drinking plenty of water will flush the toxins out of the liver and kidneys more quickly.

Cost and frequency

This treatment is not available on the NHS and costs can vary from practitioner to practitioner. An initial appointment will last approximately 90 minutes. During this a full history of your problem will be discussed before the treatment begins.

Benefits for ME and menopause sufferers

This therapy may be helpful for relieving hot flushes. As it work on the principle that blockages in the body need clearing for the organs to work effectively it should help improve your general health as well bringing it back into balance. It can also help with fatigue, stress and general aches and pains.

Reiki

What is it?

Reiki is a natural healing system which evolved in Japan. Unlike massage there is little or no pressure involved with this treatment. The practitioner may not even need to touch you and it can be performed while you are fully clothed. It is similar to laying on of hands forms of healing. It is believed to work by channelling the life energy (chi, prana or spirit) to promote well-being within the body, mind and spirit by bringing everything back into balance. You may feel the skin heating up as the healing process takes place.

Common uses

Reiki practitioners believe that this treatment restores balance to one's life and that it supports the body's ability natural ability to heal itself because the Reiki flows to the areas of need and sooths pain. They believe it is possible to heal at any level (emotional, mental, physical and spiritual).

Side-effects

The main side-effect is described as being totally relaxed and balanced although sometimes clients may experience a healing reaction. This may include feeling emotional, tiredness or a cold as a way of the body releasing toxins and unwanted stale energy. You may feel the skin heating up and even sweating in the area where the practitioner either touches you or holds their hands above your skin.

Cost and frequency

A Reiki session lasts 60-90 minutes for a full treatment. It is said that acute injuries can be helped to heal quickly but it may take longer with chronic illnesses so the number of sessions may vary from person to person. This treatment is not available on the NHS and costs can vary from practitioner but start around £30 per session although the initial session/consultation may be more.

Benefits for ME and menopause sufferers

Menopausal symptoms and ME/CFS as well as fatigue are listed among the range of illnesses which Reiki have been said to help.

Reversal Therapy, the Lightening Process, Yoga Therapy and clinics

I thought these were worth a quick mention especially as they seem to have been mentioned in the media. Although some people have reported that this has helped them enormously others have found they have had a negative effect.

Reversal therapy

This is an educational talking therapy which is used to treat anxiety, stress, trauma, post traumatic stress disorder plus the symptoms of IBS, CFS, pain management, dizziness, headaches, high blood pressure, sleeplessness, eczema and psoriasis, stomach ulcers, agitation and immune system disorders as well as emotional issues.

It believes that we can become stuck in an illness loop where we become obsessed with the illness and not being well and recovery. It helps you to understand the cause and trigger for symptoms and to be aware of the link between unresolved emotions and an increase in these symptoms. By teaching you to develop a positive mental state and stay out of a negative one it helps you to stay in the present, be more active and assertive and return to a healthy, sustainable lifestyle. It claims that by teaching people that their body needs to produce symptoms in certain illnesses so that they can understand this and work with them so that they can take appropriate action and remove the need for the symptoms.

The Lightning Process

This is one program that received considerable publicity in recent years and is a training course developed by Phil Parker. This combines gentle movements, mental exercises and meditation like techniques. It believes that when we are ill we can become stuck and stop the healing process. By changing the way we think it changes the signals sent from the brain to the body and produces physical changes/improvements in the body. A large number of their clients are people suffering with ME/CFS. It aims to teach you the tools to overcome any reasons why you are stuck in a cycle of illness. It is held over 3 days and is taught in small groups.

Yoga therapy

There are now many yoga teachers who specialize in therapy for a wide range of illness. This involves gentle movements and breathing exercises which are chosen to suit particular illnesses. Yoga has been showed to help people with ME/CFS.

Perrin technique

Dr Perrin's theory is that the sympathetic nervous system becomes overstrained due to different stress factors (physical and emotional) including allergies and infections. This believes that CFS/ME is a physical disorder which leads to a build up in the brain and spine of toxins. By helping to improve the drainage of these poisons from the central nervous system it believes it can help treat the disorder. It uses osteopathic treatments to manually stimulate the fluid movement around the brain and spinal cord. Toxins are directed out of the lymphatic system into the blood (where they are detoxified by the liver) by massaging of the soft muscle tissues.

Other clinics

When searching on the internet I also found certain clinics such as The Optimum Health Clinic which uses a range of treatments to help with ME/CFS. They are often a combination of therapies, for example, the Optimum Health Clinic uses NLP (Neuro-Linguistic Programming), the Lightning Process, Reversal Therapy, Mickel therapy, EFT (Emotional Freedom Therapy), CBT (Cognitive Behavioural Therapy), The Enneagram, Life Coaching, Hypnotherapy and self-hypnosis.

Overview

I am of the opinion that any of these may work for some people but not others. Women contacting me have found that a combination have often helped improve their health but not cure them. I myself do see an overall improvement if I have the time, money and energy to persevere with them.

Supplements

Vitamin D

We need vitamin D for calcium absorption. Vitamin D also has an important role in preventing cancer (especially breast cancer), heart disease, type 2 diabetes and osteoporosis as well as being necessary for absorbing calcium. It is also thought that good levels slow down the aging process. Low levels have been implicated in autoimmune disease (i.e. rheumatoid arthritis, lupus, inflammatory bowel disease).

Vitamin C

Vitamin C is important for preventing illness and promoting good health in the body. It is known to have a beneficial effect on the immune system as well as strengthening the blood vessels and its role as an antioxidant in the body.

It has been shown, when taken with bioflavonoid, to help reduce hot flushes. Because it helps to build up collagen, which gives skin its elasticity, it aids the prevention and treatment of vaginal dryness. It can also help prevent leakage and stress incontinence by helping to retain the elasticity in the urinary tract. Collagen is also important for good bone health.

Vitamin B

Known as the "stress vitamins" these can be beneficial if you are under pressure or stress. Symptoms of anxiety, tension, irritability and poor concentration can be due to a deficiency in these. They can also be useful if you are suffering from reduced energy levels. Taking a good B-complex is important during the menopause as it will give your adrenal glands a break (they are called into action to produce oestrogen).

Vitamin B1 (thiamine) – This vitamin is needed for a healthy functioning nervous system and normal appetite.

Vitamin B2 (riboflavin) – This vitamin is essential for healthy skin and eyes.

Vitamin B3 (niacin) – This vitamin helps maintain proper mental functioning, the nervous system and the skin.

Vitamin B6 – This vitamin is essential for the function of red blood cells and plays a role in protein and fat metabolism.

Vitamin B5 – (panthothenic acid) – This vitamin strengthens the immune system and fights infection.

Vitamin B12 (cobalamin) – This vitamin is needed for a healthy nervous system and prevents pernicious anaemia.

Vitamin B17 (amygdalin) – This vitamin is purported to control cancer.

Vitamin E

Vitamin E has been shown in clinical studies to be effective at reducing hot flushes. It is also helpful for vaginal dryness. Some researchers claim that it is more effective at reducing heart attacks than aspirin. A study in the Lancet showed that 2000 patients with fatty deposits in the arteries (arteriosclerosis) had a 75% reduction in their risk of heart attack when given vitamin E.

Chromium

Chromium helps break down sugar for use in the body and helps regulate blood pressure. This nutrient helps control insulin. Insulin's job is to remove glucose from the blood and move it into the cells. When the insulin levels are low the body stores less glucose as fat making losing weight easier. By making the cells more sensitive to insulin the pancreas does not produce as much insulin to move the glucose from the blood into the cells. Chromium is stripped away when grain is refined, as in white bread, meaning that glucose will hit the blood stream quickly affecting your blood sugar levels. Examples like this show why it is important to have good levels of chromium in the body.

Good for – Low blood sugar (hypoglycaemia)

Good sources – Cheese, meat and wholegrain

Selenium

Selenium, along with zinc, is essential to prevent the diminishing T3 hormone levels and by increasing your selenium intake it has been shown to boost thyroid function. The metabolism slows down if your T3 levels are low as it is the active thyroid hormone that burns fat.

Good for – Fibrocystic disease of the breast, breast cancer

Good sources – Meat, seafood, wholegrain cereal, brazil nuts, onions, tomatoes and cooked broccoli.

Manganese

This is needed for healthy thyroid function. It is used by the enzymes that help the body to produce the thyroid hormones.

Good for - Atherosclerosis

Good sources – Fruits, nuts, vegetables and wholegrain cereals

Bioflavonoid

Good for - hot flushes, excessive menstrual bleeding, anxiety, irritability, emotional problems, vaginal problems

Good sources – All citrus fruits (especially the pulp and pith)

Calcium

We need good calcium levels not only for our teeth, nails, hair and bones but also for healthy blood pressure and heart rhythm. Calcium is also needed for muscle contraction/relaxation, proper functioning of the nervous system and normal blood clotting.

Good for – Osteoporosis, high blood pressure (hypertension) and high concentration of blood fats (hyperlipidaemia)

Good sources – Milk and milk products, citrus fruits, green leafy vegetables, dried peas and beans.

Iron

Iron is found in the red blood cells (haemoglobin). We lose small amounts when we shed skin and through sweat and urine although the body does not really eliminate iron. We also lose iron through blood loss such as injury and menstrual periods. Women's iron levels are low until their 40s when it rises sharply although still being lower than men's. When the body has too little haemoglobin this is called anaemia. Symptoms of this are feeling tired and weak, decreased immune function and difficulty maintaining body temperature. Having too much in the body can also be dangerous causing initial symptoms of fatigue, abdominal and joint pain, weight loss, weakness. It can also cause early menopause or loss of periods, loss of libido and body hair and shortness of breath. Advance symptoms of this can be arthritis, high blood sugar and diabetes, severe fatigue, heart problems and failure, liver problems, constant abdominal pain and gray or bronze coloured skin. The only way to find out if your iron levels are correct is to have a full blood test and then be guided by your doctor.

Good for – Anaemia due to excessive menstrual bleeding

Good sources – Red meats, liver, egg yolk, green leafy vegetables, nuts and dried fruit

Iodine

This mineral combines with amino acid tyrosine which gets converted into the two thyroid hormones T3 and T4. A diet that is low in iodine is associated with an underactive thyroid (hypothyroidism) although too much iodine can actually make an underactive thyroid condition worse.

Good for – Hypothyroidism, fibrocystic disease of the breast

Good sources – Fish, seafood and seaweed

Co-enzyme Q10

Co-enzyme Q10 should not be taken by pregnant or lactating women. It can be found in foods such as meat, fish and vegetable oils. It is an enzyme found in almost every cell in the body. It is a vitamin-like substance which is important for energy production and normal carbohydrate metabolism. This is how the body breaks down the carbohydrates consumed into energy. It also plays a role in controlling blood sugar levels and lowers glucose and insulin. We become deficient in Q10 as we age which leads to depleting levels. It is claimed to play a part in neutralizing harmful oxidants which lead to cell damage and degeneration. There is no proof that it will benefit ME sufferers but some people report beneficial benefits from taking it regularly.

Ginseng

There are two main types of ginseng, Asian or Korean ginseng (*Panax ginseng*), which is more stimulating, and American ginseng (*Panax quinquefolius*). There evidence for its benefits is promising (though not conclusive) but it may help with improving mood and endurance. It may also help fight off cancer, heart disease, fatigue, high blood pressure, hepatitis C, erectile dysfunction and menopausal symptoms. It may also improve concentration and the ability to learn, albeit a modest and temporary improvement.

St John's Wort (Hypericum perforatum)

This herb has been shown to help with mild to moderate depression without many of the side effects of anti-depressants. It can reduce sleep problems and improve the quality of life but should not be taken at the same time as anti-depressants or any medication without consulting your doctor. It can cause sensitivity to sunlight if used as oil.

Valerian

Valerian is a herb used to combat insomnia and sleep disorders especially if due to mild anxiety as it has a mild sedative effect. It should not be taken by pregnant or women who are breastfeeding as it is not known what affects it may have on infants or unborn babies.

Omega 3 fatty acids

Symptoms such as dry skin, lifeless hair, cracked nails, fatigue, depression, dry eyes, lack of motivation, aching joints, difficulty in losing weight, forgetfulness and breast pain can all be blamed on the menopause but could also be connected to a deficiency in Omega 3 fatty acids, particularly if you have been trying to lose weight on a low fat or no fat diet. Taking a supplement of this can help with many symptoms of the menopause as well as lubricating the body (therefore helping with vaginal dryness). Omega 3 fats are converted in the body to have an anti-inflammatory effect on the body. Over the last hundred years there has been an 80% decrease in the consumption of Omega 3 fatty acids and we are now getting 10 times more Omega 6 fats from our diet than Omega 3.

Evening primrose oil supplements are often taken by women and are Omega 6 but you may need a supplement of Omega 3 to counterbalance this. Taking a combination of Omega 3, 6, and 9 may be good but your levels of omega 6 may be high enough to start with. A blood test can determine if you have the correct levels in your body.

Evening Primrose Oil

This is extracted from the seeds of the evening primrose flower which although native to North America also grows in Europe and some areas of the southern hemisphere. It contains vitamin F and is rich in gamma linoleric acid (GLA). It is considered a good source of prostaglandins. Although the NIH classifies it as possibly ineffective for menopausal symptoms many find that it can help counter the hormonal changes associated with the menopause. It is said to help with a wide range of symptoms which include CFS, hot flushes/night sweats, difficulty sleeping, vaginal dryness, mood disturbances, eczema, psoriasis, acne, rheumatoid arthritis, osteoporosis, high cholesterol, heart disease, breast pain, IBS, nerve damage, high blood pressure in pregnancy and obesity. It is suitable for most people but can sometimes cause nausea and an upset stomach. It can be harmful if taken with some medications as it interacts with them (such as blood thinning drugs and anaesthesia). Check with your doctor regarding any medications you may be taking.

Magnesium

Magnesium will help with symptoms such as anxiety, irritability and mood changes and is known as "nature's tranquillizer". It is also an important mineral for you bones during the menopause.

Good for – Fatigue, osteoporosis, coronary artery disease, diabetes mellitus, depression and anxiety

Good sources – Vegetables (green leafy), nuts, soya beans, wholegrain cereals

Potassium

Potassium is an important mineral because the body need it to build muscle and protein, break down and use carbohydrates, control both the electrical activity in the heart and acid-base balance as well as maintain normal body growth. It helps keep the balance of electrolytes and water (both inside and outside the cells) within the body. Having too high or low levels in the body can be serious and high levels can occur when the kidneys are not functioning correctly (these are the organs that remove any excess potassium from the body). Symptoms of your levels being too high or low can include nausea, diarrhoea, dehydration, muscle weakness or cramps, low blood pressure, frequently needing to pass water, confusion, paralysis, irritability and changes to the heart rhythm. Levels can be affected by what you eat, severe vomiting, blood pH, hormone levels and certain medications, including potassium supplements. Your levels can be measured by having a blood test.

Good for – Fatigue, heart disease, high blood pressure (hypertension), anxiety, depression

Good sources – dried fruit, bananas, orange juice, peanut butter, meat

Zinc

This plays a part in appetite control and healthy production of the thyroid hormone.

Good for - Osteoporosis

Good sources- Liver, meat, eggs, poultry, seafood

<u>Herbs</u>

Black Cohosh (Cimicifuga racemosa)

In clinical trials Black Cohosh has been shown to be effective at treating symptoms such as hot flushes and night sweats. It is also useful for helping if you suffer from anxiety and mood swings. It offers relief from symptoms without the oestrogen-like effect as it does not increase oestrogen levels. Neither does it have any effect on the cells or the womb unlike HRT which increases oestrogen and stimulates tissue in the body (including the womb and breast) increasing the risk of cancer.

Black Cohosh works as a selective oestrogen receptor modulator

(SERM). These stimulate oestrogen receptors is some parts of the body but not others like the womb and breast where over-stimulation would be unsafe. They can stimulate oestrogen receptors in places (such as the brain and bones) and block stimulation in the breast and womb. Where HRT simply replaces the hormones where SERMs target the appropriate cells. SERMs are supplied naturally in Black Cohosh and phytoestrogens.

Agnus Castus (Vitex agnus castus)

This herb is helpful during the peri-menopause as your hormones are likely to fluctuate and this helps to stabilize them. It also helps with mood swings, anxiety and tension. It is classed as an adaptogen because of its balancing effect on the hormones. It can help to increase hormones that are low and decrease those that are high by working on the pituitary gland (this is the gland that send messages to the ovary to release hormones).

Dong Quai (Angelica sinensis)

This herb has a long history of use in traditional Chinese medicine. It has been shown to help reduce hot flushes and night sweats within one month. It may also help with fatigue and disturbed sleep.

Sage (Salvia officinalis).

This is another herb which can help to control hot flushes and night sweats. It can be taken in the form of a tea to drink.

Milk thistle (Silymarin marianum)

This herb helps to improve your liver function. This is important as the liver works at detoxifying the hormones and this herb will help ease its job.

Ginkgo Biloba

Both memory and concentration declines with age in both men and women. Ginkgo biloba is a herb which has a rejuvenating effect on the brain and has shown to improve learning ability, memory and concentration in clinical trials. Studies are being made into whether it may slow down the progression of Alzheimer's disease.

Red Clover

Red clover is thought to help relieve hot flushes by regulating fluctuating hormone levels as it is a source of all the different isoflavones.

Phytoestrogens

Studies are looking at the benefits of plant hormones called phytoestrogens. Scientists began looking at the variations of menopausal symptoms and why they varied throughout different cultures where some women experience minimal and often no menopausal symptoms, also why breast cancer rates are so much lower in the Far East than the West. The UK breast cancer death rate is 6 times higher than in Japan for example.

Phytoestrogen is found naturally in certain foods like soya which contains flavonoids (genistein and daidzein). These have been shown to be chemically similar to the drugs Tamoxifen which is used to prevent recurrence of breast cancer. Although they contain weak plant oestrogens they stop more powerful carcinogenic oestrogens getting through by latching onto the oestrogen receptors in the breast. The most significant type of phytoestrogen are isoflavones which, although they have a very weak oestrogen effects compared to a woman's natural oestrogen, contain enough oestrogen to have a cumulative oestrogen effect after the menopause. Prior to the menopause they have an anti-oestrogen effect as they are competing with the high oestrogen levels. Red Clover is an excellent source of all the different isoflavones. Other sources of phytoestrogens include soya, hops, flaxseeds, alfalfa, sage, and dandelion. Phytoestrogens can also have an effect on lowering your cholesterol and can have proactive effects on heart disease, which is also important in the menopause.

You should not take any of the listed herbs if you are taking HRT, fertility drugs, the Pill, any hormonal treatment or medication unless they are recommended by a registered and experienced practitioner. Always inform your doctor if you are taking any form of alternative therapy or supplements.

Symptom	Herbal treatment
Anxiety	St John's Wort, Valerian
Breast tenderness	Evening Primrose Oil (EPO)
Circulation	Ginger, Gingko Biloba
Depression	St John's Wort
Dysmenorrhoea (pain during menstruation)	Black Cohosh
Hot Flushes	Black Cohosh, Red Clover, Sage

Insomnia	Valerian
Memory	Gingko Biloba
PMS/Mood swings	Agnus Castus, Black Cohosh

Recovery and cure versus management of ME

Many of these treatments and programs offer the promise of recovery from ME/CFS or at the very least an improvement and I as I have not attended or tried all of these I cannot recommend these or offer any opinion as to what their value is in comparison to each other. I would however suggest you take a look at the MEA survey 2010 and their results. I would say that all of these may be of benefit to some people but others have either found them unsatisfactory or worsened their symptoms. If you are thinking of trying any of these please do your research carefully as they are not cheap.

As someone who benefited greatly from receiving regular massage, reiki and reflexology treatments combined with hypnotherapy (which is relaxing in itself) I do believe that they can be beneficial but that it is difficult to afford to have them regularly, especially if you are unable to work so are on a restricted income. I have also found that I am better when I am taking a combination of supplements but that is me personally. They are not available on the NHS, even though I have been advised by my doctor that they may be helpful. Unfortunately it is expensive to be ill these days, and it can cost more to try and be better.

The Positive effects of the menopause

Not every woman's experiences of the menopause are negative. Some aspects can be positive. The absence of monthly periods can have a huge effect.

The lack of periods is the main positive that was listed by volunteers in my questionnaire. Some even went so far as to describe it as "wonderful". The absence of PMS or the associated pain of periods was seen as a big positive. Personally I found my periods extremely draining. PMS left me feeling shattered. The overall effect was that it took me about 10 days to get over each period, by the time I felt ok again I started feeling bloated and irritable and suffering from PMS. I am not at the stage where my periods have stopped completely so I can only speak about the months where I have not had one. I had a spell of 10 weeks without a period and felt great. My energy levels soared.

There have been numerous articles in the press about women who instead of suffering through their menopause have actually been given a new lease of life. If there are women out there who see this as a benefit then it stands to reason some ME/CFS sufferers may experience the same. Perhaps we don't all have to approach the menopause with a sense of dread. Yes there will be changes, and while disturbed sleep, hot flushes and mood swings might be negatives, if you are lucky enough not to experience them or they are mild, the lack of periods and the draining effect that have on our energy levels might actually outweigh them.

There are those women who feel that the menopause has given them a new found confidence. They care less what people think of them and are happier for it. The menopause is a time of change but it does not necessarily have to be a change for the worse.

Eventually the hormone levels will settle and we may feel better than we did before.

It may be that the women who contacted me were the ones experiencing difficulties and those who felt better, or at the very least no worse, did not feel the need.

The positive aspects of the menopause listed by the volunteers were

- No periods, or the tiredness and pain associated with them
- No need to worry about contraception (once menopause has passed)
- No worries about falling pregnant
- Don't feel cold anymore
- Bigger breasts! Big enough for a bra!

I am currently trying to confirm how post-menopausal women's symptoms have changed or altered as it may be that once the menopausal symptoms cease that some improvement may be seen. As yet it is too early for me to say with any certainty.

It is important to regard the menopause as another stage of life rather than the "end of life".

Things to do in your 40's and 50's

Breast Care

Check your breasts regularly for any lumps or irregularities. Remember to get regular mammograms from the age of 50. Look after your health.

Contraception

Check your contraception. As you get older you may need to change your contraception, this can be after having children or if your sex life changes. Discuss this with your doctor. You may need to continue to use contraception longer than you think!

Manage your menopause

Manage your menopause. Discuss your menopause with your doctor even before you experience any symptoms. It is best to be prepared as it may come on quicker than you think. It is best to discuss whether HRT may be right for you and what you can do to prepare yourself for this stage of your life. If you have a high risk of breast cancer or heart disease HRT may not be appropriate for you so you may have to look at other ways of managing your menopause.

Bone care

Look after your bones – Menopause is a critical time where women need to look after the health of their bones and keep osteoporosis at bay. If you cannot get enough calcium from your diet it may be necessary to take calcium supplements (please discuss this with your doctor first). Eating a healthy diet containing plenty of fruit and vegetables has been shown to lower the risk of many illnesses. It is worth remembering that you need vitamin D for your body to be able to use the calcium. You may wish to ask your doctor whether you should have a bone density scan to screen for early osteoporosis.

Watch what you eat

Remember that the number of calories you require reduces with age so it is easy for the lbs to creep on without eating any more.

Prepare your loved ones

Your symptoms may change and it is best to prepare your family for this. Rather than leave them confused by mood swings or worried that you seem to have a range of new symptoms, prepare them. The more they understand the easier it will be for all of you.

Questions to ask your doctor

Do I need any treatment for the menopause?
What symptoms should I expect?
When should I stop taking contraception?
Do I need HRT and is it right for me?
What are the risks to me of HRT?
Do I need to have a bone density screening and if so how often?
Am I at a high risk of heart disease?
Are there any tablets that I should be taking to protect my bones and heart?
Are there any medications other than oestrogen that will help relieve my hot flushes or other symptoms?
Would they recommend any natural therapies/supplements such as soya?
What type of life style changes should I adopt?
Especially considering my other conditions can they help me set

up a sensible exercise routine?

If you are on medication already will I be able to continue to taking them?

Strictly speaking the menopause is the time when your periods have stopped. Most doctors will consider you in the menopause when you have not had a period for 12 months. You may well experience symptoms in the time leading up to the menopause. This is known as the peri-menopause. Even if you are still having your monthly periods but are experiencing symptoms your doctor can perform a blood test to determine your hormone levels. This will tell you whether you are entering the menopause or not. It is best to be prepared and if you don't understand keep asking for them to explain it until you do.

Relationships – Partners, children and friends

I believe that when you are ill relationships, whether that is with family or friends, become more important so you don't become isolated. It can be a real problem because you can find that you just don't have the energy to communicate with them or even if you want to sometimes. Friendships, and even relationships, can fall by the wayside. You may not have the energy to stand up for yourself let alone express your true feelings. Alternatively you might not feel you have the luxury of considering everybody else's feelings. You might not be able to give the support back to your loved ones that you feel you should which can intensify feelings of being useless.

Being a carer for anyone with a long term illness is hard. It is difficult for anyone to understand how we actually feel especially since everyone gets tired at times. Trying to convey that this illness doesn't leave you feeling "a bit tired" but mentally and physically exhausted can be another frustration for the sufferer and at times incomprehensible to their family and friends.

There can be a tendency for people around you to think that you'll feel better next week or that you might snap out of it for Christmas. Even worse they might consider it is "all in your mind". Both you and they may desperately want the person you once were back, when that may not be possible. Inevitably we all change through life, some relationships and friendships run their course anyway but when we are forced to change and reprioritize our lives because of illness these relationships have no choice but to change.

It is a good idea for family to read as much as they can about your illness and accompany you to the doctors so they can ask any questions regarding your health. There is plenty of information to be found on websites such as www.meassociation.org.uk/ and www.actionforme.org.uk/

It may also be helpful to consider some form of counselling for either you as a couple or as a whole family. In the MEA survey where carers rated what options helped to provide the best care for their patients visiting a counsellor rated 38%. Sometimes it is harder to talk to someone close to you than someone who is impartial. Your partner or family may benefit from talking to someone neutral too. An illness can be a big change for everyone and some may need more help than others adapting to it. Use everything at your disposal to make this transition and acceptance of these changes as easy as possible because stress will only exacerbate your symptoms which will not help anyone.

The MEA survey also highlighted the benefits that carers felt they gained from carers support groups as well as the need in some cases for respite care for their patients and training in patient handling.

It is important that carers make time to pursue their own hobbies and interests. There are groups where advice can be given for them as well. A happy carer makes for a happier patient.

It is a difficult balance between staying involved in family activities and using all your energy to keep everyone else happy. Almost every volunteer reported that stress had a negative impact on their ME symptoms.

I think that the responses I have included say it best, so here are some examples for you.

Do you feel your relationship with your partner has suffered because of your illness?

45%   Yes
20%   No
30%   No comment
10%   Not in a relationship

"Yes, very much."

"No really my partner has always been very supportive."

"My previous long-term partner did not understand at all when I got ME and was thoroughly unsupportive. I had already had chronic fatigue symptoms for some years, which I and everyone else ignored, so he thought I was making a fuss about nothing much."

"My last partner and I got together when I already had ME, so he was quite understanding and accepting at first, especially as I was in a relatively good phase when I met him. My menopause coincided with his own health problems which was not a good combination and resulted in us splitting up."

"It altered my relationships by making me unable to keep up physically or in conversations. It has altered new relationship because of how I see myself – I am not sure of who I am or what I do now compared to before. How I think I should or could be is different from how I currently function and how someone new sees me"

"Yes, some days I literally can't do a thing and I feel I am a burden and boring."

Have you had any relationship breakdown because of your illness?

40%   Yes although 20% said it highlighted existing problems

20%   nearly but we go through it

40%   No

20%   Only with friends

"It had a devastating effect on my marriage and ultimately caused it to breakdown."

"Only with friends."

"Some friendships."

"It came close some years ago but we worked through it."

"I should have left the partner I was with when I got ME anyway, the ME just highlighted the necessity to do so."

"Very nearly coming to that."

"The relationship I was in when I started being ill suffered and broke down."

"Being ill showed up all the weak areas in our marriage, we probably would have split up anyway but the ME didn't help."

Do you feel that your relationship with your children has suffered because of your illness?

33% No

33% Yes

33% It changed it

"I don't think it suffered but it changed. My son was 19 and off to Uni and my daughter was 14-15. I think it enabled them to grown up quicker and become more self-confident."

"They were only 4 and 8 and have grown up with me having ME."

"They can't remember me not being ill."

"Because I couldn't do any sporty activities they have chosen less physical activities and hobbies themselves so we could do them together."

"I think me being ill has made us closer."

Do you find yourself doing activities that they want because you don't want them to miss out?

75% Yes

8.3%   No

8.3%   Depends

8.3%   Have illnesses themselves

"Yes, all the time."

"I feel I don't have a life for me as every little bit of energy I have I spend trying to please my partner/kids/grandchildren/brothers and sisters."

"I feel selfish if I say NO to them and then do something I actually want to do"

"I have to prioritise my time and I am often left with no energy to

do what I want, then I feel resentful"

If you choose to spend your energy doing something you want to do, do you feel guilty?
72%   Yes
14%   No
14%   Not so much now

"Not so much now but I used to"

"I honestly never do anything I want to do as I am too busy trying to please others. I feel I have so little time to give so when I am able I feel I have to help them or spend time with them."

"Yes often because they assume that I don't want to spend time with them"

"It can cause arguments when I choose to do what I want because I have no energy left to do things with them. It's a no win situation, if I keep them happy I miss out and if I do what they want I miss out on my interests."

Who is your primary carer?
22%   I am my own carer
22%   Partner
5%   Friends
5%   Home help
There were 39% of volunteers who did not answer this question. This could mean they are well enough not to need help or that they manage on their own. This compares with The MEA survey 80% of carers came from within the family.

What role does your partner take in assisting you in your everyday living?

44% cooking and household chores

44% shopping

44% driving

33% moral support

22% tells me to rest

22% doesn't

11% financial

11% gardening

Only 53% of volunteers answered this question. This is not a simply question to answer because what one family considers a normal everyday amount of help isn't necessarily the same as another family. For every wife whose husband is a "new man", there will be another married to a "caveman". The MEA survey rated carers main roles as 91% daily living (cooking, cleaning), 86% shopping and errands, 78% accompanying to appointments, 60% help with mobility outside the house, 32% personal care, 28% mobility in the house and 25% other.

How does he cope?

11% Just gets on with it

22% They find it hard

11% Is already a carer

22% Throws himself into work

22% Is very supportive and understanding

11% Doesn't believe it

22% frustrated but practical

50% did not answer this question at all but those with helpful partners often listed more than one way.

"He just ignored it and pretended it wasn't happening. Ultimately

the relationship broke down."

"He learnt to alter his expectations. I've been ill so long that this is just our lives now."

"...threw himself into work but that may have been helpful as he could escape the illness."

"He still wants the 'me' I was and would rather be doing things with me than go out and do activities without me."

"He finds it restrictive at times which frustrates him. He wants us to do things together and sometimes is hurt that I have no enthusiasm because of my energy levels."

"The relationship broke down eventually so I guess he didn't."

"I encourage him to still take part in his interests and hobbies. I will rest then so we can still do some more sedate activities that we both enjoy."

What types of family activity are easiest?

33%   Watching TV

33%   Trips out (art galleries, museums) where I can take my time and sit in the cafe

33%   Eating out and cinema

33%   Short duration, low key activities

22%   Talking

11%   Playing with younger children

11%   Watching others enjoy themselves

11%   Don't do family activities anymore

What activities do you no longer do?

42%   Any sport/physical activity

33%   Holidays

33%   Socializing

17%   Shopping

8%   Playing family games

8%   Cooking for large family get gatherings

The absence of sport came as no surprise but the main thing we women miss are holidays, socializing and shopping.

What roles do your children take in assisting you in your everyday life?

25%   Driving me places/pushing wheelchair

25%   Bringing me shopping

25%   Cooking meals

25%   Small jobs around the house

25%   Generally supportive

13%   Personal care

13%   Stimulation and laughter

50%   Are ill themselves or live away

Do you feel guilty asking for their help?

62.5% Yes or sometimes

37.5% No

Those who didn't feel guilty either felt that they didn't need help or that it was a mutual thing. Included in those who said yes explained that when their children saw how much help was needed they wanted to help and the sufferers had learned to accept this.

Have your children had to adapt to your illness?

75%   Yes

37.5% They are grown up

25%   Have their own illnesses

There were only a small number of responses to this question but out of those no-one said a straight NO.

"My eldest son was upset to begin with (he was 8 at the time) and hated me using a wheelchair. The younger one just took it all in his stride"

"My children can't remember a time when I wasn't ill so it was just the way we lived our lives. They learnt that there were times when I needed to rest more than other Mums or that at times I needed them to be quiet. They learnt to look out for and after each other more"

"There were times when I couldn't deal with having their friends around as much but I think they coped ok. I had to try not to over-compensate by spoiling them in other ways because I felt guilty."

How has your illness changed your relationship with your partner on a practical level?

"We don't go on holiday or for days out as I can't walk far and I'm a hindrance to others. Jobs at home are now shared, though at the beginning of my ME I was unable to do anything and my husband had to give up work to look after me and the children."

"He couldn't accept that I had changed and I needed him to look after me for a change. Instead he had to work even harder to support the family and it caused stress even if he wouldn't talk about it. He simply ignored it as much as possible, eventually we split up"

"I have already had a failed marriage because I couldn't do things

with him so he found someone else who could, with my new partner I feel I am pushing myself to try to do as much as can housework wise but then I crash and burn. Holidays are something I have not managed to do with him yet."

"Not really. I use a wheelchair when I leave the house and we have just taken that on holiday. I always want to go somewhere warn though."

"It has ruined it."

"It had a devastating effect on my marriage and ultimately caused it to breakdown."

"Having the use of a wheelchair made holidays possible. We chose city holidays so that when I am resting my husband could go and explore on his own. He had to take over the weekly shop but the development of the internet made it possible for me to do the monthly shopping."

"I do find that I try to rest when he is out and then rush jobs so he doesn't see how much rest I need. I feel useless most of the time so I don't like him to see how exhausted I get. If he thinks I have been doing jobs he won't feel as if he is the only one doing the housework."

"We have lost our favourite social pastime of eating out due to ME and food intolerances."

"Holidays are very limited now."

"I have to be more selfish now and make sure I do things that I

want to do. This means saying no to everyone including my partner at times. Choosing between what I want to do and spending time with him or the children makes me feel guilty but if I didn't I would have no energy to do the things I enjoy and life would be unbearable."

Do they resent this?
50%   Yes
50%   No

Do you feel that your partner *really* understands your illness?
29%   Yes
57%   No
14%   Not completely/more than he used to do

Has your illness placed additional financial pressure on your family?
80%   Yes
20%   No
I won't even attempt to try and unravel the mysteries of the benefits system in the UK let alone abroad but will advise anyone struggling to seek advice on what they are entitled to claim. Financial stress and worries will not help your ME/CFS symptoms or smooth the way for an uneventful menopause. Money may not be able to buy your health but lack of it can make it worse. Carers rated benefits advice at 55% in the options to provide better care for your patient part of the MEA survey which is not surprising considering the amount of paperwork involved and the complexity of applying for benefits.

Reassessing your life and time management

Pacing is vital for anyone suffering from ME/CFS but it is a good idea to reassess this from time to time. As this is a fluctuating illness, changing sometimes on a daily basis, we also need to be prepared to constantly change the way we live our lives and react to it. The MEA survey found that the therapy for general management that most people felt the MEA should recommend to the NHS was pacing and activity management (81.7%), followed by dietary advice (83.8%), alternative therapies (59.6), counselling - not CBT (49.5%), CBT (27.7%) and lastly GET (24.1%).

Many years ago I read several books by Shirley Conran looking at managing your time better. All of her "Superwoman" and "Down with superwoman" books are brilliant for everyday life and parts are particularly useful for anyone with ME. It is only through my research that I have discovered that she too is an ME sufferer and has been for many years. She believes that the secret to being a superwoman is elimination. This is not specifically written for women with illness but for people who want to manage their time more efficiently and don't want to spend their entire life cleaning etc.

The menopause can be another change in your life and your symptoms and much of what she suggests may be relevant if fatigue is something which is affecting you badly. The information in this chapter can be used to make life easier at anytime of your life but if is worth reiterating for women going through the menopause. For those who have suffered for years I apologize if it seems like I am going over old ground but truthfully when was the last time you seriously looked at how you are dealing and managing your illness? Perhaps it might be worth doing it now when you are facing even more changes.

You have to learn to come to terms with any type of long-term illness and ME/CFS are no exception. While we may all hope for a miracle cure to come along so that we can go back to the "real you" there is a need to accept that your life has changed. This does not mean that it has ended or there is nothing to look forward to or that you will never be able to live a fulfilling life. Everyone has limitations put on them in life, be it laws, rules or commitments. It is just you might now have more. Feeling too tired to be able to function in normal life at times can be frustrating, demoralizing and depressing. There may be times when you actually long to do jobs that you would previously avoided, times when you wistfully remember spending the whole weekend spring-cleaning the house but now it feels exhausting to wash up your own cup. The mental effect can be as devastating as the physical. This is why pacing yourself and learning to reorganize your life to work with this illness is so important. Becoming depressed will only make everything feel worse and you feeling helpless, quickly becoming a vicious cycle which will hamper any recovery at all. It is worth remembering that by nature this illness is a fluctuating one. The fact that it fluctuates means that if you feel really bad right now you might feel a bit better soon.

When you read stories about other sufferers who have recovered and are leading full lives or achieving wonderful things it is easy to feel that it's ok for them, they must be the lucky ones and perhaps they are. The prospect of being able to complete a marathon might seem about as achievable as a trip to the moon but there are stories of sufferers who have overcome this illness and have been able to complete the full 26 miles. Being a fellow sufferer I am certainly not prescribing to the "it's all in your head" attitude to which I frequently want to scream "if it was all in my head don't you think I would choose to be well? I want to be better, I want to be able to do everything I used to do" but I do know how easy it is to feel so hopeless and helpless when I am exhausted just by getting out of bed and making it down the stairs. I also know that wallowing and feeling sorry for my self achieves nothing, changes nothing except making me more miserable. Staying positive and taking positive action puts me back into control to some degree.

"A real achiever isn't a woman who can do anything, but a woman who avoids doing too much. She knows her limitations and sticks happily within them." – Down with Superwoman (Shirley Conran)

Know your best times

There is a big difference between being in the middle of a relapse and how you feel when your illness has stabilized but knowing when your energy levels are at their highest and lowest can help.

Try keeping a record of your energy levels and rate it as to how good or bad you feel. You will usually find that there are certain times of the day when you feel more alert than others. By realizing when you are at your best or worst you can begin to reorganize your life. Rate your energy into 4 categories –

a) Your Prime energy time. This is when you feel you are at your best.
b) Your Good energy time. This is when you can do things but not as much as during your prime time.
c) Your OK energy time. This is when you can do routine tasks but no more.
d) Your Low energy time. This is where you are barely functioning. You can watch TV but not much else.

Once you have assessed which are you best times you can start to work with your illness rather than against it. You need to fit you day around your energy levels rather than the other way around. It is important not to use your prime energy levels (a) to sleep and to avoid doing too much during your good (b) and ok (c) times. Keep your prime time for doing something positive and productive. Before we look at budgeting your time we need to look at what is going to fill it. Don't spend all your energy on planning though as it can be tiring but neither should you prepare your lists when you are exhausted because you will miss things off.

LISTS

What you want to do - The "me" list

Now make another list, just for you. Put on it everything you *want* to do. Do not put what you feel you should do, only put on it things that you want to do. There doesn't have to be any reason for it other than you want to do it. If you enjoy gardening, put it on there because you want to do it not because the grass is 2ft high. It doesn't matter if you feel you haven't got time to fit it in or will never have the energy to do it. Make it a bucket list of all the things you want to do in your lifetime. Nobody else needs to see this list it is only for you.

Once you have your list you can split it down into smaller lists. What do you want to do in the next 3 months, 6 months, and the next year? What do you want to do within the next 5 and 10 years? Look at how you might achieve these things. Look at which are most important to you and try to break them down into small steps to make it possible. We will come back to these lists later in the chapter.

What needs doing - The "to do" list

Divide this up into "things that are urgent and need doing" and "things that need doing that aren't that important". Please don't start to feel overwhelmed at this point or start thinking that you will never be able to get them all done.

Dissect and delegate

The next step is to look at each job on your to do list and see if each one can be broken down into smaller jobs. It will make your list look much longer but it is important to do this. If, for example, you take a mundane job like cleaning the bathroom it can be broken down into lots of small jobs like this.

- Put dirty towels into wash
- Put clean towels on the rail
- Clean the sink
- Clean the bath
- Clean the toilet
- Clean the shower
- Vacuum and wash the floor

There are 7 jobs on this list. You could choose to do one each day or clean the sink after you have had your morning wash, or take the clean towels into the bathroom on your way for a lie down. Perhaps you can delegate the larger jobs such as cleaning the bath and/or shower or to wipe and bleach the toilet each day. If you live with your family make sure that they are doing their share. Ask them to look at the list of broken down chores and ask which they think they can do. By breaking the jobs down into small bits it is amazing how much more you can all achieve. Getting everyone to take even 10 minutes to do a job or two and get them done can reduce the list quickly.

Look carefully at these to do lists and ask if the items are really that important. Ask yourself "what would happen if I just didn't do them?" and you might find that the answer is ... nothing! There are always going to be plenty of jobs that must be done, such as paying your utility bills so you still have heat and lights but do the curtains really need washing or can they wait another week or even months?

Take a look at the jobs on the list that you *hate* doing. Does it really need to be done? Can someone else, who doesn't mind, do it instead? Can they do it quicker and easier than you? We all have those jobs that we leave and try to push to the back of our minds hoping they will go away. They can prey on your mind and you can guilty feel them nagging away at you. This is a complete waste of your energy, especially when you have so little. Feeling that you have a whole host of things that you haven't done can bring you down and being depressed can be tiring in itself so get it done and off the list, even if it means paying someone to do it. Remember that your energy levels can soar if you are doing something you enjoy but plummet if it is something you hate. Think carefully, is there anything that you can do without so you can pay someone to do that particular job which will also free you up to achieve something more enjoyable?

If you start the morning feeling overwhelmed by the mountain of things to do and you just don't know where to start then stop. Stop, put the kettle of and sit down. Spend half an hour if necessary to write a list of what *must* be done today. Then start with something easy and quick, that way you won't lose heart and feel that you can't do anything.

It is important to remember that other people might not do jobs in the same way or to the same standard as you. You need to remember to let go and perhaps relax your standards. It is better that someone do the job, even if it is to a lesser standard, than it not be done at all.

Budgeting your time

Look and decided when you have your prime energy levels. This is the time for you to tackle jobs that you really *have* to do or activities that you really *want* to do. If you choose to sleep or watch TV then you are wasting your time. This is the time for you to be productive. Do be careful not to get carried away and do too much though. Take regular breaks.

It might be easier to pick the jobs that you need doing but you don't really like first to get them out of the way. Alternatively try to do one job you hate followed by one you enjoy. You might find it more satisfying to take one job you hate and several small jobs (with breaks between if needed) so that you can physically see them being ticked off. Clearing items off your list will make you feel like you have achieved something. You can use this time to go out and see friends and socialize so you can really enjoy it but make the most of this time.

Make sure that you make time to do things on your "me" list. If you would rather be reading than cleaning then alternate 10 minutes cleaning and 10 minutes reading. If it is a good book you will be amazed to discover how much you can get done just to get back to it. It might be that this is all you can manage during your prime time or this might be something you can do in your good (b) or ok time (c).

When you reach your low energy time, or the (d) category, use this time to rest. It might be that you should lie down and sleep or do less tiring activities such as watching TV. Do not plan to be productive during this time.

When looking at any activity ask yourself –

- Is it necessary? Does it really *need* doing?
- Where is the best place for this task or activity
- Is now the best time to do it? Is there a better time?
- Am I the best person to do this job? Can someone else do it with far less effort? Have they got the time to do it?
- What is the best way to do this activity?

Remember that you can choose what you put into your plan. You can choose what to put onto today's list. You can also change it if you are having a bad day. You can say no without feeling guilty. You have every right to say no, even if it is just because you don't feel like it. Do not feel pressured by what you feel you *should* or *ought* to do. Instead look at what you *have to* and what you *want to* do.

Plan your day to avoid rushing and organize tasks and where possible combine them. Make sure you pace yourself and allow adequate time for rest especially after difficult tasks. Try to alternate light and heavy tasks to avoid becoming overtired and prioritize tasks as what has to be done and what can be left for a day or a week.

Another way is to simply allow yourself a set amount of time to work at your list. It might be 10 minutes, it might be half an hour, but try to get as many jobs as possible done in that time and then stop and put your feet up. You might decide that is enough for today or that you can do another session. Either way you can be happy that you have achieved what you aimed to do which was work for a set amount of time. You may leave the rest of the list until another prime time either later in the day or even tomorrow but you will be able to see what you have achieved and be able to use this as a guide for what you can realistically expect to achieve another time. You may be able to do some lighter jobs during your b or c times to reduce the list.

If the item on the list is recreational such a meeting friends then you can still set yourself time limits if it helps. Tell them that you would love to see them for half an hour, or an hour even but stick to it so as to not overtire yourself and leave when you are feeling good. Your memory then will be of having enjoyed your time rather than the exhaustion you felt because of it.

Housework

Housework is part of life but the first thing you have to do is learn to let go. I am not promoting living in chaos but you don't *have* to have a spotless house. There is no rule that says that your home should look like a show home. You must decide what is more important to you. Do you want to use your energy for doing things you enjoy or trying to maintain a standard you had before you became ill? If having an immaculate home *is* more important, then fine, if not relax and let go a bit.

- Break jobs down into smaller ones
- Delegate or pay people to do difficult jobs
- Combine as many jobs as you can

Tips for the kitchen

- Try to sit down when preparing food or washing up
- A dishwasher saves putting pressure on your hands (particularly when scrubbing pans). It is also a job which can be delegated to someone else. If you live alone table top dishwashers save bending.

- Simple planning. When preparing a meal carry everything to the area you are working at in a basket or bowl to save making more trips than necessary.
- Make use of aids such as electric tin openers if you have problems with your hands. (take a look at aids for disabled people to see if any will help you)
- Make things easier for yourself and buy frozen vegetables. It's a simple way to have a healthy varied diet with the minimum of effort.
- Double up. It can often take very little effort to make double the quantity so you have enough for 2 or more meals. You can freeze any extras for days when you do not have as much energy.
- Slow cookers are a brilliant way of producing healthy warming stews with the minimum of effort.
- Change the way you use potatoes. Jacket potatoes, cooked either in an oven or microwave, are easier to make than mashed. Chips and roast potatoes can be bought frozen and just put in the oven.
- Microwave rice. Rice can be cooked quickly in the microwave, some do not even need taking out of the bag.
- Salad and fruit can be bought ready washed and cut. It costs more but is ready to eat.
- It doesn't have to be done all at once. You can peel the potatoes in the morning, cut the vegetables at lunch time and cook at tea-time.
- Have a supply of paper plates etc so on a really bad day you can just throw them away and avoid the need to wash up
- It isn't going to kill you if you survive on sandwiches or beans on toast for a day. Some days it might be simpler to take the easy option.
- Halogen cookers, rice cookers, slow cookers and microwaves can all save you time and effort. Look at how they might save you time and energy. Use them if they will but if you can't think they

will fit into your style of living then don't waste your money, they will only end up as something else to clean.

Shopping

- Make use of smaller trolleys or motorised trolleys for disabled people
- Always have a list otherwise you will come back without the thing you need most
- Internet shopping. Shopping can be tiring and most supermarkets will, for a fee, pick and deliver your shopping for you. Personally I find that the length of time it takes me to process my order on line just as tiring as going to the supermarket but you may find this an easier option
- Accept help with your packing. If you are disabled most supermarkets will help you take your shopping out to the car
- Supermarkets may also deliver your shopping to your door. Some make a charge for this and others will do it for free if you spend over a certain amount. They will pack your shopping, arrange a delivery time slot and drop it off so all you have to do it put it away
- Ask family or friends to shop for you
- Schemes such as dial-a-ride will allow you to book transport to and from the supermarket for a fee if you don't have your own transport
- Remember that shopping can be tiring so factor this in when you are budgeting your energy

Around the house

- Use duvets not sheets and blankets

- When washing/changing beds split the loads up. You could change the pillow cases one day, the sheets the next and the duvet cover on another.
- Consider buying a comfortable chair with a high or raised seat to help with getting up and down
- Minimise the effects of tasks by maintaining the correct posture when sitting and standing, lifting properly and taking the weight off your feet when resting
- If you use the internet invest in a laptop table on wheels (the feet can slide under the sofa or the bed) or a laptop tray. This means that you can sit with your feet up while using them
- Use the hands free option on the telephone if your hands hurt
- Buy clothes that do not need ironing and if you have to iron sit down to do it
- Have a vacuum upstairs as well as downstairs to saving having to carry it up and down. Also have it fitted with a long flex so you don't have to keep bending to plug and unplug it
- Telephone sockets. Try to have one fitted upstairs so you don't have to get down stairs to answer it. Alternatively make sure you have a charged cordless phone which you can take with you
- Have 2 washing baskets, one for lights and one for darks then you don't have to sort it before washing

Make use of the telephone and internet

- Most banks now offer online banking. Sometimes you may even get a better deal by having an online account. You can pay your bills etc from home without going out
- You can purchase almost anything these days from home. It can be clothes to electrical goods. Catalogues may sometimes be more expensive but you can try them on at your leisure and return if they don't fit meaning you don't have to struggle in changing rooms which can be tiring

- Buying online and through comparison sites can save you money
- If you regularly use the computer for writing there are now programs which can type as you speak such as Dragon software

Clothes

- Buy clothes that are do not need ironing or dry cleaning
- Wear slip on shoes or sandals
- Elasticised trousers needn't be unfashionable and are easier to get on and off than jeans
- Avoid belts which can be fiddly
- Choose tops that are pull on rather than ones with small buttons or fastenings
- Use bed socks and gloves if you are susceptible to cold
- Using a tumble drier can save you having to bend and stretch to hang washing on a line (it also lessens the need for ironing)

Out and about

- If you have difficulty getting about you might consider a mobility scooter. There are expensive but are available for hire. Obviously walking is good exercise if you can manage it. There is a danger that if you have a mobility scooter that you may opt to use it all the time and stop walking anywhere outside therefore it is imperative that you use this type of aid when you need it and not just because you have it. Please ensure that you know how to control it before you speed merrily about on one. There have been a significant number of cases where people are being injured by disabled peoples running into them on their scooters. Just because you can go at high speeds doesn't mean that you should.
- Make use of walking aids such as walking sticks or frames if you need them

- If you feel unsteady ask someone to go with you. I frequently grab hold of my husband's arm when we are out to help me keep my balance
- Plan rest stops when travelling and try to avoid places where you have to queue

General

- Keep warm. Cold can exacerbate your symptoms
- If you are sensitive to light and noise during a bad spell investing blackout curtains and consider earplugs. Double glazing can block out some noise from outside so if you are ill shut the windows (do remember that fresh air is good for you though so open them when you are not in the room resting)
- Evaluate each task to find the simplest and least trying way of doing them so they will leave you energy to activities that your enjoy
- Implement routines for other people in the house so everyone knows what they need to do and allowing you to do the things that you can

Hobbies and activities

Gardening

- Raised beds can save bending
- Have a comfortable seat that you can sit in to take regular breaks
- Use a stool or chair in the green house or potting shed
- Use long handled tools to avoid bending

Brain activities

These can help to keep you mentally active

- Crosswords

- Word search
- Sudoku
- Online courses – There are often long and short courses available to further your education or just for personal interest with personal tutors that you can contact for help and advice. These can often be done at your own speed so you can take breaks if you are feeling unwell

Games to enjoy with the family

Sometimes you may feel that you are losing out on spending quality time with your loved ones but there are games that you can play without having to over exert yourself.

- Scrabble
- Boggle
- Chess
- Draughts
- Othello
- Connect four
- Trivial pursuit
- Who wants to be a millionaire
- Card games

And numerous other games.

Hobbies that are not too strenuous

Listed below are a range of hobbies that you could enjoy without too much physical effort

- Writing
- Art – painting and drawing
- Needlework – embroidery, cross-stitch, tapestry

- Knitting or crochet
- Stamp collecting
- Photography
- Scrapbooking
- Computer games
- Watching TV or films
- Listening to music

Hobbies that require a bit more energy

- Learning to play an instrument
- Singing – it could be karaoke or joining a choir
- Walking
- Exercise classes such as yoga and tai chi (see chapter on exercise for more details)
- Gardening

The menopause is another time for change. Mentally as well as physically we can sometimes feel that we are at a crossroads in our lives and the menopause can affect us in the same way that we may have felt when we first became ill. Our symptoms and energy levels may have changed. If you are well enough to work you may decide that now is the time for a change of career. Old hobbies or activities may have become redundant, family commitments may have altered, even the time when you have most energy may have changed so it can help to reassess what changes you need to make your life work better for you. Life is not static, therefore the way we live may have to change as well.

Personal experiences and advice from other sufferers going through the menopause

"When the menopause first happened it was very frightened as I did not anticipate going through such huge changes at such a young age. I felt I was maybe having a breakdown emotionally as I felt so low and I was incapacitated with overwhelming fatigue. Sex was extremely painful and this was also very scary as I felt I had nobody to discuss this with."

"I have a daughter with Aspergers Syndrome who needs a lot of listening times and can talk for hours about her problems! I find I don't have the same patience or concentration now and have to take regular breaks or just stop her talking when I can't take anymore in. Now that she's 18, I worry much more about the future and this can impact on my relationship with my partner. To be honest, I worry that I am possibly getting Alzheimer's as there are days when I fell disorientated and disconnected and need a lot of silence in order to regain some degree of normalcy. I have helped with the Brownies for years but recently find the noise of the girls chattering unbearable. It is embarrassing when I can't remember all their names and annoying when the leaders joke about my poor memory. It's hard to have a sense of humour about this subject ..."

"Since the menopause my ME/CFS has been worse, I struggled to keep working, taking holidays at least once a week using all my holiday entitlement for sick days instead of getting a holiday, eventually it caught up with me and I couldn't get out of bed so had to go on the sick, my body aches, migraines and exhaustion became unbearable"

"In 1999, aged 47, I experienced a significant worsening of the ME I had already had for 10 years. My ME started suddenly and was very severe when I first got it, then after a couple of years I had a particular form of treatment and made a big improvement, not recovery, but was much better. Then as peri-menopause started I found my stamina reduced and I could no longer do specific things – accelerate in the swimming pool (I am a good swimmer and at times I have been able to swim further than I can walk), drive a car nor attend conferences. I think it is partly because of my information-processing capacity has dropped quite significantly. And obviously I have lost general stamina; although I can still swim a bit I must go slowly and carefully and rest a lot more than before, or I will come out of the pool feeling much worse. In addition, the treatment I had had which had helped me so much no longer had the same beneficial impact and I had to find alternative ways of supporting my health (none of which were ever as effective)."

"I am a happier person."

"I developed ME at about the same time as I got the menopause about 8 years ago. I am now 57. When I was very ill what seemed to happen was I would feel terrible (extra terrible!) usually in the evening for up to an hour and then I would get a hot flush and feel a bit better. Every time I had a hot flush I felt worse. Now I am not so ill (although still have ME and am house bound with very little energy), I am STILL getting hot flushes but they are not as bad. I don't the terrible ill feeling but I often get a sort of anxious feeling before hand and they drain all my energy so I have to go and lie down. I have wondered over the years how much ME has exacerbated them as when I have relapses the flushes seem much worse. Or whether some of the flushes have been due to ME and not menopause? I have considered HRT (and still sometimes do)

but I am so hopeless with drugs that I haven't dared. Sometimes it feels like I am going to have hot flushes forever! Also since I haven't experienced ME before the menopause, I don't know if it would have been worse but I am hoping that when it finally goes perhaps I will feel a bit better and have more energy."

"Get all the help you can. Get a good mainstream specialist and invest in alternative therapies."

"I thought I was losing my mind. My emotions were all over the place, crying one minute the boiling with rage the next. I felt like someone had taken me over and I had no control and I didn't know why. Physically I felt better for several months as I didn't have a period. I had far more energy but was wound up like a spring. When I went to the doctors' blood tests showed that despite being only 40 years old I was going into the menopause so was given HRT which gave me breast cysts so I stopped and opted for natural alternatives. I am back to having periods and the mood swings are less severe but I am now constantly tired. I'm hoping that once my periods stop for good I might get some of those energy levels back but without the mood swings."

"Take each day as it comes. Talk to each other about each family members feelings. Work with ME; don't fight it. Definitely pace yourself. Don't be afraid to say, No I can't manage that activity"

"Listen to your body, spend time (weeks or months in necessary) learning how the illness affects them, ask for help when you feel you need it and not to beat yourselves up because there are things you can no longer do. The sooner you accept the illness and its restrictions the sooner you can start looking for a recovery plan. It took me 10 years to realise that I did not have to spend the rest of my life as an invalid and another 5-6 to achieve complete recovery."

"My relationship, that I had when I started being ill, suffered and broke down. I am a very different person now I am ill. Obviously what I can do is very different, my boyfriend and social circle were high level rowers. I was also a much stronger person than I am now which altered the dynamic with that and subsequent boyfriends. It altered my relationships by making me unable to keep up physically or in conversation with my previous friends. Then it has altered new relationships because of how I see myself – I am not as sure of who I am and what I do as I was before. And I am much less happy with how I look because with so little ability to do anything about it now due to lack of energy. How I think I should or could be is different from how I currently function and how someone new sees me. That has cause problems too."

"My ME is made much worse in the days leading up to and during my period by making me much more tired, I cannot do the same amount of activity as when I am not having a period due to the fatigue and also more muscle and joint pains especially in my legs."

"I don't have anyone to ask for help. Friends and relatives really just do NOT understand what it is like to have zero energy when they are used to me leading such a full life prior to the ME. I was a company director, had a hectic social life and was a regular at the gym. Everyone still invites me to parties and it seems that no matter how many times I try to explain my illness they just seem to think that maybe next week I'll be over it and back out clubbing. I am normally a very positive person but it isn't easy with this condition."

"For me hormonal change has been like going to hell in handcart but at least it clarified for me what I was really suffering from. I think the menopause affected me not just from the point of view

170

of hot flushes and night sweats disturbing my sleep and causing further stress on my body but also the loss of progesterone and subsequent oestrogen dominance seemed to make my allergies and intolerances much worse. I have some allergy neutralisation therapy and nutritional supplements which have helped but there is still considerable room for improvement and my life is very restricted. At the age of 62 I find going on holiday or even just out for the evening virtually impossible. Shopping is difficult and even reading for too long can worsen symptoms drastically. My social life, as well as my career, has been totally ruined but now I have a home help and am a member of a support group which has been very important to me."

"The menopause has played very much a part alongside ME. In fact I would say that it has been difficult at times to know what symptoms are because of the ME and those relating to the menopause. I've had ME 9-10years and I couldn't really say when my menopause started (I am now 55). My periods became heavier and heavier and eventually I needed a hysterectomy. Recovery was slower than a "normal" person and I went into rapid intensive menopause symptoms. The worse was the hot flushes. I did try taking some soya based alternative tablets which helped somewhat. Still with no bleeding my energy levels have improved. I still hot flushes 3 years on and maybe other symptoms of the menopause or is it the ME? It's hard to know for sure."

"I'm not sure when I first became ill because it always seems to have been with me in one form or another (I'm 66). 6 years ago I was diagnosed with ME and I am still struggling with very debilitating fatigue and am largely housebound. I have tried all sorts of things but to no avail. One thing that stands out to me is that when I look back on my life and at all my periodic symptoms are that they all tie in with how I am now. The only difference I can

see is that previous to this "attack" I have always got better. This time I was post menopausal and I have not got better. I have mentioned this to several doctors and none of them seem to know so your interest in this really struck a chord."

"Sometimes I feel resentful that I am limited because of the fatigue and pain. I've had it for so long now that I'm not sure I can remember what it is like to be normal. I work a few hours a week and am shattered by it (which feels pathetic because I am exhausted for a whole day after 3 or 4 hours work). I feel like I have to justify why I can't do more because I look well. I try and hide just how tired I am from everyone. I try to stay positive but it's not always easy because people don't seem to understand how this tired is different from them being tired after work because this doesn't go away. It feels like I am wasting my life spending all my energy doing the stuff that has to be done (and failing to keep up with that) and being too exhausted to enjoy trips out or things I want to do. Hot flushes are just exacerbating the issue. I feel so weak and unwell afterwards that all I want to do is lie down."

"I had my last period in 2005 and my hot flushes started then. In the beginning it was worse when I had a hot flush. They would make me feel really unwell, dizzy weak nausea and like a wave of weakness came over me. I can still feel like this but not as much. I have insomnia with night sweats and one of the main factors of NOT feeling well and having ME symptoms next day is lack of sleep and in this way the menopause affects me greatly. When I have hot flushes at night I feel really unwell and even faint unlike other people who do not have ME. I have all the other traits of Menopause and ME, foggy brain, lack of concentration, bouts of mild depression, anxiety etc (which one is which I do not know). I feel that when my hot flushes and night sweats stop then my ME may improve."

"It started to feel as if the menopause and the ME were interacting and it became hard to tell what was causing what, but I really believe one was exacerbating the other e.g. lots of thrush. I was sore and dry even when washing, horrendous sweats with a masculine and pungent odour and completely lethargic. My skin was much drier and thinner and lines were more obvious. I was sleeping during the day to compensating for hardly sleeping at night. I did some reading about oestrogen and found it actually supports the very challenges with which ME presents! Devastated. I'm amazed I'm not depressed. Life has changed dramatically for me. I could feel sorry for myself but I believe my life has more meaning and these challenges only serve to make me focus more on my own needs. This does not feel selfish, more self-honouring. Reflexology and shiatsu have helped me a lot so has a good diet and supplements. I have learned to love myself and accept/integrate, not lie down to my difficulties."

"I have wondered over the years how much ME has exacerbated my symptoms as when I have relapses the flushes seem much worse. Or whether some of the flushes have been due to ME and not the menopause? I started the menopause 8 years ago when I was 49. When I was very ill I would feel extra terrible for up to an hour and then have a hot flush after which I would feel a bit better but getting worse with each one that followed. I am STILL getting hot flushes although not as bad and although I don't get the terrible feeling I get a sort of anxious feeling before hand and they drain me of all my energy so I have to go and lie down. I haven't experience ME before the menopause so I don't know if it would have made it worse but I am hoping that when it finally goes perhaps I will feel a bit better and have more energy. Sometimes it feels like I am going to have hot flushes forever."

"Get as much help and support from the NHS as is available in your area. Join a support group if there is one locally. Never underestimate the importance of pacing and avoid over doing things when you are having a good spell – the constant cycle of boom and bust is not good for our condition. Don't ignore problems that cause tension and try to approach things in a non judgemental way, both with yourself and those are important to you. If you are having a bad day, let your family know – don't expect them to always realise. Loosen or cut ties with those who refuse to accept your condition or who suggest "it might all be in the mind"!! Try and keep your stress levels (if possible) to a minimum and learn to say NO to requests that may lead to a worsening of your symptoms. Try not to lose hope as there is always the possibility of getting better."

"Read as much as you can about the changes and how they affect you. Explain to your family/partner and friends how the menopause can affect you behaviour and mood. Talk through difficult situation and ask for support and understanding when you feel it's lacking. Talk with your GP or nurse about various treatments, including alternative treatments. Look after your bones."

Conclusion

Obviously when I started this project I had hoped to come up with a clear answer, for myself if nothing else, of how my symptoms would be affected. I wanted to know what to expect but as with the nature of this illness it is not that simple.

Some women definitely experienced a worsening of their symptoms, others experienced the exact opposite. The responses were not clear cut as to a yes you will or no you won't. Perhaps if I had received more response it would have presented a clearer picture but I was reminded during a discussion with my doctor that the human body is not that easy.

He reassured me that even with tested and recommended medication what works for one person won't work for another. He commented that it was refreshing to find someone who accepted this rather than wanting a magic cure.

When we look at the variety of symptoms and the variations in severity it is logical that the effects of the menopause should also be also be varied and different from woman to woman. Those without ME/CFS are affected differently so why should we all be the same?

Having written and published this book I have since re-edited it slightly, mainly hoping to correct and spelling errors (blame self-editing and brain fog!). I am currently sending out a simpler revised survey to both women going through the menopause and post-menopausal women to try and ascertain if any exacerbation of ME symptoms pass with time when we enter the post-menopausal stage of our lives. I will then be able to add that information to this book.

I hope that at some point the medical community will look into what symptoms we should expect and how best to handle them but until then I will continue to collect as much information from the women who are going through the menopause themselves.

At times the results may be inconclusive but I can only tell you what has been reported to me. Hopefully though their experiences may help you, or at least comfort you, that you are not alone.

Abbreviations

CBT	Cognitive Behavioural Therapy
CFS	Chronic Fatigue Syndrome
DVT	Deep Vein Thrombosis
EFT	Emotional Freedom Therapy
EPA	Eicosapentaenoic Acid (Omega 3 fatty acids)
EPO	Evening Primrose Oil
FSH	Follicle Stimulating Hormone
GET	Graded Exercise Therapy
GLA	Gamma Linoleic Acid
HRT	Hormone Replacement Therapy
IBS	Irritable Bowel Syndrome
LH	Luteinising Hormone
ME	Myalgic Encephalomyelitis
MEA	ME Association
NIH	National Institute of Health
NLP	Neuro Linguistic Programming
PMS	Pre Menstrual Syndrome
POF	Premature Ovarian Failure
PTSD	Post Traumatic Stress Disorder
PVFS	Post Viral Fatigue Syndrome
SERM	Selective Oestrogen Receptor Modulation
TATT	Tired all the time
WHI	Women's Health Initiative

Sources and useful contacts

Women's Health Handbook – Dr Miriam Stoppard
Natural Solutions to the Menopause – Marilyn Glenville PHD
Hormones or Natural Alternatives – Jan Clarke
The Menopause without weight gain – Deborah Waterhouse
Complete essential Oils - Julia Lawless
Everyday Aromatherapy – Karen Philip
M.E. – Dr Anne Macintyre
Living with M.E. the chronic/post-viral fatigue syndrome
by Dr Charles Shepherd
Alternative therapies – Daily Mail 25/10/12 Anna Hodgekiss
http://www.nlm.nih.gov/medlineplus/medlineplus.html
www.marilynglenville.com
http://ods.od.nih.gov
www.webmd.boots.com
www.cdc.gov
www.hearthealthywomen.org
www.Hpathy.com
www.livestrong.com
www.superskinnyme.com
www.about.com
www.ehow.co.uk
www.arthritiscare.org.uk
www.painconcern.org.uk
www.outsiders.org.uk
www.spokz.co.uk
www.fpa.co.uk

Action for ME, P O Box 2778, Bristol, BS1 9DT
www.actionforme.org.uk/
Tel 0845 123 2380

ME Association, 7 Apollo Office Court,
Radclive Road, Gawcott,   Bicks, MK18 4DF
Tel 0844 576 5326
www.meassociation.org.uk
Email: meconnect@meassociation.org.uk

CHROME (Case History Research on ME),
3 Britannia Road, London, SW6 2HJ
Tel 0207 736 3511
Chrome.prime.cfs.org/

National ME Centre and Centre for fatigue Syndrome,
The National ME Centre, Long Term Conditions Centre,
Gubbins, Lane, Harold Wood, Romford, Essex. RM3 0AR
www.nmec.org.uk
Tel 01708 378050
Email: nmecent@aol.com

The CFIDs Association of America,
PO Box 220398, Charlotte, NC 28222-0398,
704-365-2343
www.cfids.org/
Email: cfids@cfids.org

The National CFIDS Foundation,
103 Aletha Road, Needham, MA 02492
Tel (0781) 449-3535
www.ncf-net.org/
Email: info@ncf-net.org

ACUPUNCTURE

British Medical Acupuncture Society
BMAS House, 3 Winnington Court, Northwich, Cheshire,
CW8 1AQ
Tel 01606 786782
www.medicalacupuncture.co.uk
Email: admin@medical-acupuncture.org.uk

BMAS, Royal London Hospital for Intergrated Medicine,
60 Great Ormond Street, London, WC1N 3HR
Tel 020 77137437
Email: bmaslondon@aol.com

British Acupuncture Council, 63 Jeddo Road, London,
W12 9HQ
Tel 020 8735 0400
www.acupuncture.org.uk

ALLERGIES
The British Allergy Foundation, Deepdene house,
Bellegrove Road, Welling, Kent, DA16 5PY
Tel 0208 303 8525
www.allergyfoundation.com

Allergy UK, Planwell House, LEFA Business Park,
Edington Way, Sidcup, Kent, DA14 5BH
Tel 01322 619898
www.allergyuk.org
Email: info@allergyuk.org

Action Against Allergy, PO Box 278. Twickenham, TW1 4QQ
Tel 020 8892 2711
www.actionagainstallergy.co.uk
Email: aaa@actionagainstallergy.freeserve.co.uk

ALTERNATIVE & COMPLEMENTARY MEDICINE

The British Holistic Medical Association,
5 Sea Lane Close, East Preston, West Sussex, BN16 1NQ

The Institute for Complimentary and Natural Medicine,
Can-Mezzanine, 32-36 Loman Street, London, SE1 0EH
Tel 0207 922 7980
www.icnm.org.uk

AROMATHERAPY

International Federation of Aromatherapists,
20A The Mall, Ealing, London, W5 2PJ
Tel 0208 5672243
www.ifaroma.org

Bach Flower Remedies
The Bach Centre, Mount Vernon, Bakers Lane,
Brightwell-cum-Sotwell, Oxon, OX10 0PZ
Tel 01491 834678
www.bachcentre.com

BACK PAIN

National Back Pain Association, 16 Elmtree Road,
Teddington, Middlesex, TW11 8ST
Tel 0845 130 2704
Helpline Tel 02089775474
www.backcare.org.uk

CHINESE MEDICINE
Register of Traditional Chinese and Herbal Medicine, Office 5,
1 Exeter Street, Norwich, NR2 4QB
www.rchm.co.uk
Email: herbmed@rchm.co.uk
Tel 01603 623994

CHIROPRACTIC

The British Chiropractic Association, 59 Castle Street,
Reading, Berkshire, RG1 7SN
Tel 0118 950 5950
Email: bca@publicasity.co.uk
www.chiropractic-uk.co.uk

HEALING

The Healing Trust, 21 York Road, Northampton, NN1 5QG
Tel 01604 603247
www.thehealingtrust.org.uk

HERBALISTS

The National Institute of Medical Herbalists, Clover House,
James Court South Street, Exeter, EX1 1EE
Tel 01392 426022
Email: info@nimh.org.uk
www.nimh.org.uk

HOMEOPATHY

The British Homeopathic Association, Hahneman House,
29 Park Street West, Luton, LU1 3BE
Tel 01582 408675
Email: info@britishhomeopathic.org
www.britishhomeopathic.org

The Society of Homeopaths, 11 Brookfield, Duncan Close,
Moulton Park, Northampton, NN3 6WL
Tel 0845 450 6611
www.homeopaths-soh.org/

HYPNOTHERAPY

The General Hypnotherapy Register, PO Box204,
Lymington, SO41 6WP
www.general-hypnotherapy-register.com/

The General Hypnotherapy Standards Council,
PO Box 204, Lymington, SO41 6WP
www.ghsc.co.uk
Email: admin@gneral-hypnotherapy-register.com

MIND (The National Association for Mental Health),
Granta House, 15-19 Broadway, Stratford, London,
E15 4BQ
Tel 0300 123 3393 (information line)
www.mind.org.uk
Email: contact@mind.org.uk

THE Seasonal Affective Disorder Association, PO Box 989,
Steyning, BN44 3HG
Tel 0181 9697028
Email: contact@sada.org.uk
www.sada.org.uk

SAMARITANS
Freepost RSRB-KKBY-CYJK, Chris, PO BOX 90 90, Stirling,
FK8 2SA
Tel 084579 90 9090
www.samaritsns.org/

MIGRAINE

The Migraine Action Association, 4th Floor, 27 East Street,
Leicester, LE1 6NB
www.migraine.org.uk/
Tel 0116 275 8317

The Migraine Trust, 52-53 Russell Square, London,
WC1B 4HD
Tel 0207 631 6970
www.migrainetrust.org
Email: info@migrainetrust.org

NATUROPATHY

The General Council and Register of Naturopaths,
1 Green Lane Avenue, Street, Somerset BA16 0QS
Tel 01458 840072
www.naturopathy.org.uk/

OSTEOPATHY

The General Osteopathic Council, 176 Tower Bridge Road,
London, SE1 3LU
Tel 0207 357 6655
Email: contactus@osteopathy.org.uk
www.osteopathy.org.uk

OSTEOPOROSIS

The National Osteoporosis Society, Camerton, Bath,
BA2 0PJ
Tel 0845 450 0230 (helpline)
www.nos.org.uk
Email: info@nos.org.uk

PAIN RELIEF

The British Pain Society, Third Floor, Churchill House,
35 Red Lion Square, London, WC1R 4SG
Tel 0207 7269 7840
Email: info@britishpainsociety.org
www.britishpainsociety.org

PHYSIOTHERAPISTS

Chartered Society of Physiotherapy, 14 Bedford Row, London,
WC1R 4ED
Tel 0207 306 666

PREMENSTRUAL SYNDROME

The National Association for Premenstrual Syndrome,
41 Old Road, East Peckham, Kent, TN12 5AP
Tel 0844 8157311
www.pms.org.uk/

REFLEXOLOGY

Association of Reflexologists, 5 Fore Street, Taunton, Somerset,
TA1 1HX
Tel 01823 351010
www.aor.org.uk

RELATIONSHIPS

RELATE, Herbert Gray College, Little Church Street,
Rugby, Warwickshire, CV21 3AP
Tel 0300 100 1234
www.relate.org.uk

SLEEP

The British Snoring and Sleep Association, Chapter House,
33 London Road, Reigate, Surrey, RH2 9HZ
Tel 01737 245638
Email: info@britishsnoring.co.uk
www.britishsnoring.co.uk

Index

O

Osteoporosis	16, 36, 52, 55, 56, 89, 124, 127, 128, 129, 136, 137, 138
Oestrogen	10, 12, 13, 15, 26, 27, 30, 37, 40, 42, 44, 48, 52, 53, 54, 55, 56, 58, 67, 71 74, 75, 86, 95, 96, 97, 99, 121, 129, 131, 137, 171, 173
Ovaries	11, 12, 15, 74, 95, 98
Omega 3 Fatty Acids	81, 126, 127

P

Perrin	120
Peri-menopause	11, 12, 13, 27, 130, 138, 168
Pre-mature menopause	12, 53
Post Menopause	13
Pre-menopause	11
Panic Attacks	36, 37, 38, 109
Pelvic Floor	49, 50, 51
Progesterone	10, 15, 74, 75, 95, 171
Protein	27, 31, 75, 80, 81, 123, 128

R

Reflexology	2, 115, 133, 173
Reiki	2, 117, 118, 133
Reversal Therapy	118, 120
Red Clover	131, 132
Relationships	2, 3, 68, 71, 139, 141, 170

S

Sex	44, 62-68, 100, 136, 167
Sleep Disorders	6, 15, 30, 71, 126
Selenium	123
St John's Wort	39, 126, 132
Sage	107, 101, 131, 132
Swimming	37, 91, 93, 168

About the author

The author has been living with ME since her late 20's.
She lives and works as a writer and hypnotherapist in
Bridlington, East Yorkshire.

Me not ME!

I remember the days when I used to run,
Just as a way of life and not just for fun.
It's a distant memory of what used to be,
Before I stopped being me and became just ME.
How can I tell you how tired I feel?
When it feels like a dream and doesn't feel real.
Whenever I walk my legs feel like lead,
The only friend I enjoy seeing these days is my bed.
I ache and I hurt and I'm in constant pain.
My brain feels like mush and I think I'm insane.
I want to be normal. I want you to see.
I'm not just an illness, I'm not just ME.
I know I'm not being just lazy and idle,
And at times I'm depressed and feel suicidal.
My brains full of fog and my head hurts from thinking,
I hate lots of noise and I can't tolerate drinking.
I was outgoing, that used to be me,
Now I'm just a woman who lives with ME.
My body needs me to be gentle and kind
And if I am careful I usually find,
I can have good days, weeks, sometimes more,
When I can walk not crawl on the floor.
I can walk, I can think, I can do all of that,
And I only need one afternoon nap.
Still people say "but you always seem tired"
I want to scream "This is not the life to which I aspired."
I want my life back. I want to be me,
Not a horrible illness, I'm not just ME."
My legs won't support me. I hit the ground with a bump.
My balance deserts me and I walk like a drunk.
I want to walk and know I'll not collapse,
To do what I want without fear of relapse.
I hate this illness that you call ME,
But I'm literally too tired to find the real me.

(From My Teacher is a Witch and other Poems)